ADOLESCENT MEDICINE: STATE OF THE ART REVIEWS

Adolescent Sexuality

GUEST EDITORS

Susan L. Rosenthal, PhD

Margaret J. Blythe, MD

December 2007 • Volume 18 • Number 3

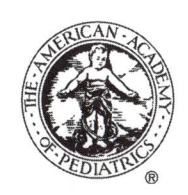

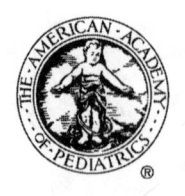

ADOLESCENT MEDICINE CLINICS:
STATE OF THE ART REVIEWS
December 2007
Editor: Diane E. Beausoleil
Marketing Manager: Linda Smessaert
Production Manager: Shannan Martin

Volume 18, Number 3
ISBN 978-1-58110-287-1
ISSN 1934-4287
MA0433
SUB1006

Copyright © 2007 American Academy of Pediatrics. All rights reserved. No part of this publication may be reproduced or transmitted in any form or by any means, electronic or mechanical, including photocopying, recording, or any information retrieval system, without written permission from the Publisher (fax the permissions editor at 847/434-8720).

Adolescent Medicine: State of the Art Reviews is published three times per year by the American Academy of Pediatrics, 141 Northwest Point Blvd, Elk Grove Village, IL 60007-1098. Periodicals postage paid at Arlington Heights, IL.

POSTMASTER: Send address changes to American Academy of Pediatrics, Department of Marketing and Publications, Attn: AM:STARs, 141 Northwest Point Blvd, Elk Grove Village, IL 60007-1098.

Subscriptions: Subscriptions to *Adolescent Medicine: State of the Art Reviews* (AM:STARs) are provided to members of the American Academy of Pediatrics' Section on Adolescent Health as part of annual section membership dues. All others, please contact the AAP Customer Service Center at 866/843-2271 (7:00 am–5:30 pm Central Time, Monday–Friday) for pricing and information.

EDITORS-IN-CHIEF

VICTOR C. STRASBURGER, MD, Professor of Pediatrics, Division of Adolescent Medicine, University of New Mexico, School of Medicine, Albuquerque, New Mexico

DONALD E. GREYDANUS, MD, Professor of Pediatrics, Michigan State University; and Pediatrics Program Director, Kalamazoo Center for Medical Studies, Kalamazoo, Michigan

GUEST EDITORS

SUSAN L. ROSENTHAL, PhD, Division of Adolescent and Behavioral Health, Department of Pediatrics, University of Texas Medical Branch Children's Hospital, Galveston, Texas

MARGARET J. BLYTHE, MD, Department of Pediatrics, Indiana University School of Medicine, Indianapolis, Indiana

CONTRIBUTORS

BETH A. AUSLANDER, PhD, Division of Adolescent and Behavioral Health, Department of Pediatrics and Sealy Center for Vaccine Development, University of Texas Medical Branch, Galveston, Texas

DEVON BERRY, PhD, University of Cincinnati College of Nursing, Cincinnati, Ohio

FRANK M. BIRO, MD, Division of Adolescent Medicine, Department of Pediatrics, University of Cincinnati College of Medicine, Cincinnati Children's Hospital Medical Center, Cincinnati, Ohio

MARGARET J. BLYTHE, MD, Department of Pediatrics, Indiana University School of Medicine, Indianapolis, Indiana

JANE D. BROWN, PhD, School of Journalism and Mass Communication, University of North Carolina, Chapel Hill, North Carolina

MARINA CATALLOZZI, MD, Heilbrunn Department of Population and Family Health, Mailman School of Public Health, Columbia University, New York, New York; College of Physicians and Surgeons, Columbia University, New York, New York

JENNIFER CHRISTNER, MD, Division of Child Behavioral Health, Department of

Pediatrics, University of Michigan Medical School, Ann Arbor, Michigan

SIAN COTTON, PhD, Departments of Family Medicine and Pediatrics, Institute for the Study of Health, University of Cincinnati College of Medicine, Cincinnati, Ohio

PAM DAVIS, MD, General Pediatrics, Department of Pediatrics, University of Michigan Medical School, Ann Arbor, Michigan

ABIGAIL ENGLISH, JD, Center for Adolescent Health & the Law, Chapel Hill, North Carolina

ALISON J. LIN, MPH, Heilbrunn Department of Population and Family Health, Mailman School of Public Health, Columbia University, New York, New York

MARY A. OTT, MD, Section of Adolescent Medicine, Department of Pediatrics, Indiana University School of Medicine, Indianapolis, Indiana

MARISSA RAYMOND, MPH, Heilbrunn Department of Population and Family Health, Mailman School of Public Health, Columbia University, New York, New York

LYNN REW, EdD, RN, AHN-BC, FAAN, Department of Nursing, University of Texas, Austin, Texas

VAUGHN I. RICKERT, PsyD, Heilbrunn Department of Population and Family Health, Mailman School of Public Health, Columbia University, New York, New York; College of Physicians and Surgeons, Columbia University, New York, New York

DAVID S. ROSEN, MD, MPH, Division of Child Behavioral Health, Department of Pediatrics, University of Michigan Medical School, Ann Arbor, Michigan

SUSAN L. ROSENTHAL, PhD, Division of Adolescent and Behavioral Health, Department of Pediatrics, University of Texas Medical Branch Children's Hospital, Galveston, Texas

RICHARD RUPP, MD, Department of Pediatrics, University of Texas Medical Branch, Galveston, Texas

OWEN RYAN, MPH, MIA, Heilbrunn Department of Population and Family Health, Mailman School of Public Health, Columbia University, New York, New York

JOHN S. SANTELLI, MD, MPH, Heilbrunn Department of Population and Family Health, Mailman School of Public Health, Columbia University, New York, New York

MICHAEL G. SPIGARELLI, MD, PhD, Division of Adolescent Medicine, Cincinnati Children's Hospital Medical Center, Cincinnati, Ohio

VICTOR C. STRASBURGER, MD, Department of Pediatrics, University of New Mexico School of Medicine, Albuquerque, New Mexico

ADOLESCENT SEXUALITY

CONTENTS

Preface x
Susan L. Rosenthal, Margaret J. Blythe

Puberty 425
Frank M. Biro

> Puberty consists of interrelated biological changes and occurs at a time when the individual also encounters cognitive and social changes. In this article we examine our current knowledge regarding the onset of puberty, the sequence and timing of puberty, and medical issues and physiologic changes that may arise with pubertal maturation. Figures included demonstrate the sexual maturation stages and interrelationships between the various parameters of puberty.

Understanding Sexual Behaviors of Adolescents Within a Biopsychosocial Framework 434
Beth A. Auslander, Susan L. Rosenthal, Margaret J. Blythe

> In this article, adolescent sexual behavior is discussed within a biopsychosocial framework. Prevalence rates for both coital and noncoital behaviors are presented, and trends in coital behaviors are noted over time. Special attention is paid to the role culture plays in the development of sexual behaviors. The discussion includes prevalence rates and trends of pregnancies/births and sexually transmitted diseases among adolescents and the impact of these outcomes for both adolescents and their offspring.

Development of Intimate Relationships in Adolescence 449
Marissa Raymond, Marina Catallozzi, Alison J. Lin, Owen Ryan, Vaughn I. Rickert

> This article examines adolescent intimacy through a developmental lens. As they age, adolescents develop the relational skills necessary to gain independence from their parents and form intimate relationships with friends and romantic partners. This article details how adolescents' intimate relationships expand from parental connections to encompass friendships, dat-

ing, and sexual activity during progressing stages of development. Finally, clinical implications for adolescent health care practitioners for promoting intimacy and healthy relationships are suggested.

Parental Influences on Adolescent Sexual Behaviors 460
Richard Rupp, Susan L. Rosenthal

Parents play a significant role in the sexual development and behaviors of their children. Parental monitoring and supervision are important avenues for keeping adolescents from risky situations and activities while the teen develops responsible decision-making skills. A supportive relationship between the parent and adolescent is important for enhancing communication and supervision. In this article we discuss programs that were designed to improve parenting skills to decrease adolescent sexual risk behaviors.

Religiosity, Spirituality, and Adolescent Sexuality 471
Sian Cotton, Devon Berry

There are many individual, family, and cultural factors that influence the development of healthy sexuality in adolescents. One factor that is less often described but may play a role is religion/spirituality. Adolescents' religious/spiritual belief system or the cultural religious context within which they are raised may impact their attitudes or beliefs about having sex before marriage, decisions about the timing of coital debut, or contraceptive practices. In this article we will define the terms "religiosity" and "spirituality"; highlight the key scientific literature on the relationships between religiosity, spirituality, and adolescent sexual health outcomes (eg, coital debut, contraceptive practices), including describing why religiosity/spirituality may be related to these outcomes; and briefly discuss programs/clinical implications for integrating these findings into clinical practice.

From Calvin Klein to Paris Hilton and MySpace: Adolescents, Sex, and the Media 484
Jane D. Brown, Victor C. Strasburger

In the absence of effective sex education at home or school, the media have become important sources of sexual information for adolescents in the United States. Mainstream media inundate teenagers with sexual images and innuendoes. In the most recent content analysis of American primetime TV, more than three-fourths of the shows had sexual content; yet less than 15% contained any references to responsible sexuality, abstinence, the risk of pregnancy, or the risk of sexually transmitted infections. Dozens of studies attest to the power of the media to influence teenagers' beliefs and attitudes about sex. Three longitudinal studies have all found that adolescents exposed to more sexual content are more likely to begin having sexual intercourse earlier than their peers who see or hear less about sex in the media. The media could become part of the solution as well as part of the problem – if there were more responsible portrayals of human sex and more widespread advertising of birth control products.

Adolescent Sexual Orientation 508
Michael G. Spigarelli

Sexual orientation has been defined as the patterns of sexual thoughts, fantasies, and attractions that an individual has toward other persons of the same or opposite gender. Throughout childhood and approaching adolescence, children try to understand their own sexuality and sexual orientation in the context of the society in which they live. Typically, this attempt to understand first occurs in thoughts of a sexual nature and later through actions, usually before sexual orientation is clearly defined. How these experiences are handled, by the individual and close friends and relatives, helps to define how an individual views and accepts their sexual orientation ultimately as an adult.

Sexual Health of Adolescents With Chronic Health Conditions 519
Lynn Rew

Adolescents with various chronic health conditions face the same challenges associated with physical, cognitive, emotional, and social changes that are characteristic of this developmental stage. Many of these adolescents face unique challenges related to their health conditions that add to the complexity of sexual maturation and reproductive function. This article is an overview of the health risk behaviors of adolescents with chronic health conditions and how these conditions relate to various aspects of sexual health. Suggestions for anticipatory guidance of these young people are also addressed.

Relationship Violence in Adolescence 530
Alison J. Lin, Marissa Raymond, Marina Catallozzi, Owen Ryan,

Vaughn I. Rickert

> Previous experience with violence or a deficit in interpersonal skills may lead to violence in adolescent relationships. In this article we focus on various forms of interpersonal violence (bullying, sexual harassment, coercion, and relationship violence) that adolescents may experience and pay special attention to risk factors, help-seeking behaviors, and sequelae.

Office-Based Interventions to Promote Healthy Sexual Behavior   544
Jennifer Christner, Pam Davis, David S. Rosen

> In this article we describe adolescent-friendly office policies, address approaches to developmentally appropriate counseling in the office setting, and outline the medical needs of the sexually active patient. Specific topics include optimizing office effectiveness and efficiency, counseling regarding appropriateness of and readiness for sexual intimacy, immunizations, prevention of sexually transmitted infections, and pregnancy and addressing sexual orientation and sexual violence.

Approaches to Adolescent Sexuality Education   558
Mary A. Ott, John S. Santelli

> The purpose of this review is to examine evidence in support of comprehensive and abstinence-only approaches to sexuality education for adolescents. In this article we review the effectiveness, medical accuracy, and ethical concerns related to different approaches to sexuality education.

Sexual and Reproductive Health Care for Adolescents: Legal Rights and Policy Challenges   571
Abigail English

> Laws developed over the past half century have significantly improved adolescents' access to essential sexual and reproductive health care. These laws allow many adolescent minors to give their own consent, protect confidentiality, and provide financial support for the care. The consent requirements for adolescents to receive health care are contained primarily in state court decisions and in statutes known as "state minor consent laws," which are based on either the minor's status or the services sought. Confidentiality protections for adolescents' health information are contained in these minor consent laws, in the federal medical privacy regulations known as the "HIPAA Privacy Rule," and in state medical privacy laws. Other signif-

icant laws include statutes providing for the emancipation of minors, court decisions delineating the mature minor doctrine, regulations protecting adolescents' access to confidential family planning services in publicly funded programs, and court decisions interpreting the constitutional right of privacy. Special considerations apply to consent and confidentiality questions pertaining to family planning, contraception, and pregnancy-related care for minors. In addition to the explicit provisions of state minor consent laws, many of the most important considerations are articulated in court decisions based on the constitutional right of privacy and the confidentiality requirements that are part of the federal Title X Family Planning Program and Medicaid.

Index 582

Preface

Adolescent Sexuality

Sexual feelings and behaviors are a part of everyone's life; yet, we struggle as health care providers, as parents, and as a society to know how to provide an environment that supports the psychosexual development of our adolescents. Everyone has the same goal, which is to guide adolescents into adulthood knowing how to make healthy sexual decisions. However, reaching that goal is a complicated process that becomes embedded in our cultural values and political systems. Although most of our adolescents are learning how to have intimate relationships, are making good decisions, and are avoiding sexually transmitted infections and mistimed pregnancies, it is easy to focus only on those adolescents who make poor decisions.

For this issue we assembled the leading national and international experts to provide readers with a broad knowledge base and a balanced, scientifically based discussion. The authors reviewed the scientific literature regarding adolescent development and behaviors and discuss efforts to help adolescents in the office and through sexual education programs. Adolescent sexuality begins with an understanding of pubertal development and the range of adolescent sexual behaviors. Sexual development and decision-making takes place in the context of families and peers and is influenced by our spiritual beliefs. Unfortunately, although most adolescents have the opportunity to explore intimacy and sexuality in a safe context, not all of them do, and some experience coercion and violence. It is critical that we remain sensitive to that possibility so that we can help to prevent its occurrence or treat the sequelae. When one initially considers adolescent sexuality, one tends to think of heterosexual relationships in physically healthy adolescents. However, not all adolescents are heterosexual, and other adolescents are questioning their sexual orientation or gender identification. As medicine advances, we have greater numbers of adolescents who are facing mastery of adolescent developmental tasks, including sexuality, in the context of chronic illnesses. Regardless of health status or health care needs, adolescents' access to comprehensive sexual and reproductive health services is significantly affected by an array of federal laws as well as laws that vary from state to state.

As we worked with the authors on this issue, we were struck by both the wealth of knowledge they have assembled on adolescent sexuality and the opportunities presented for the research community to learn even more. In addition, we were

Copyright © 2007 American Academy of Pediatrics. All rights reserved. ISSN 1934-4287

left with a sense of awe of the gift that adolescents give us when we have the chance to be a part of their lives as they explore this complex but important part of their physical and emotional world. We hope that you are left with a similar sense and a desire to pursue these topics as a clinician and/or researcher.

Susan L. Rosenthal, PhD
Division of Adolescent and Behavioral Health
Department of Pediatrics
University of Texas Medical Branch Children's Hospital
Galveston, Texas

Margaret J. Blythe, MD
Department of Pediatrics
Indiana University School of Medicine
Indianapolis, Indiana

Puberty

Frank M. Biro, MD*

Division of Adolescent Medicine, Cincinnati Children's Hospital Medical Center, Department of Pediatrics, University of Cincinnati College of Medicine, 3333 Burnet Avenue, Cincinnati, OH 45229, USA

Puberty is a biological construct of interrelated changes that incorporate several systems, which include linear growth, changes in body composition, maturation of the adrenal axis, reactivation of the hypothalamic/pituitary/gonadal (HPG) axis, and the achievement of the ability to reproduce. As adolescents encounter the biological changes associated with puberty, they also go through cognitive and social changes.

From a cognitive perspective, the majority of adolescents progress from concrete to formal operational thought, which is also known as abstract thinking. Other processes associated with these cognitive changes include egocentrism, overthinking, and apparent hypocrisy. As Hume commented, "Reason is . . . the slave of the passions"[1]; for adolescents, these observations are especially salient. Dahl defined what is termed "cool" cognition (calm) and "hot" cognition (emotionally charged) in adolescents.[2] There are physiologic underpinnings to these observations. Portions of the frontal lobe, such as the dorsolateral prefrontal cortex, an integral area of the brain for impulse control, mature later than most other areas of the brain.[3] In stressful situations, when there may be a prominent affective contribution, the adolescent brain may be less likely to modulate the affective component on decision and action (ie, hot cognition).

Psychosocial issues with which the adolescent must deal include independence, establishment of adult self-identity/sexual identity, and engagement in plans for self-sufficiency. As noted above, these social changes occur at the same time as important changes in the brain, and changes in body composition, as well as adrenal and sex hormones. Adolescence, then, may be considered as a paradigm of chronologic age interacting with biological change.

---

*Corresponding author.
E-mail address: frank.biro@cchmc.org (F. M. Biro).

"PRIMARY" PUBERTY AND THE ONSET OF "TRUE" PUBERTY

There is a functioning luteinizing hormone-releasing hormone (LHRH) pulse generator and HPG axis in the third trimester in life. The HPG axis is turned off in the first year of life, initially through negative feedback from sex steroids, and subsequently through inhibition by neuropeptides. γ-Aminobutyric acid is an important component of this inhibition, and reduction of γ-aminobutyric acid inhibition is felt to be a critical factor in disinhibition of the LHRH pulse generator. Leptin, a peptide hormone produced by adipocytes, seems to function as a permissive factor, but not a trigger, in the onset of puberty. One trigger that has been suggested is kisspeptin 1, a member of the rhodopsin family of G protein–coupled receptors. Mutations in GPR54 are associated with hypogonadotropic hypogonadism in humans and mice, and it is proposed that kisspeptin regulates release of gonadotropin-releasing hormone at the level of the hypothalamus.[4] During the late prepubertal period, there is increased amplitude and frequency of LHRH pulses that initially occur at night; ultimately, this leads to increased secretion of follicle-stimulating hormone (FSH) and LH, and the onset of true (adolescent) puberty.

Although these terms have been used interchangeably, the accepted definitions for adrenarche, pubarche, thelarche, gonadarche, and menarche are as follows:
Adrenarche: The activation of the adrenal medulla for the production of adrenal androgens, which typically occurs before the onset of puberty.
Pubarche: The appearance of pubic hair.
Thelarche: The appearance of breast tissue.
Gonadarche: The activation of the gonads by FSH and LH, which are pituitary hormones.
Menarche: The age of onset of the first menstrual period.

Several studies have used menarche as a substitute for onset of puberty, because age at onset of puberty and age of menarche are correlated.

SEQUENCE AND TIMING OF PUBERTY

Several important parameters to consider when discussing pubertal maturation include stage (sequence), age at onset (timing), and rate of progression (tempo). Sequence and timing seem to have a greater impact on physiological and psychological changes. Sequence is defined by the sexual maturity ratings, also called "Tanner stages," after James Tanner, a British physician.[5] Figures 1 through 3 demonstrate the sexual maturity ratings. These photographs were published by van Wieringen and provide an excellent illustration of the breast and pubic hair stages.[6] Stages range from 1 (prepubertal) to 5 (adult). Figures 1 through 3 provide a description of each stage. Tanner and others have defined genital stages on the basis of maturation of the scrotum and penis. Many clinicians and researchers have commented on the lower

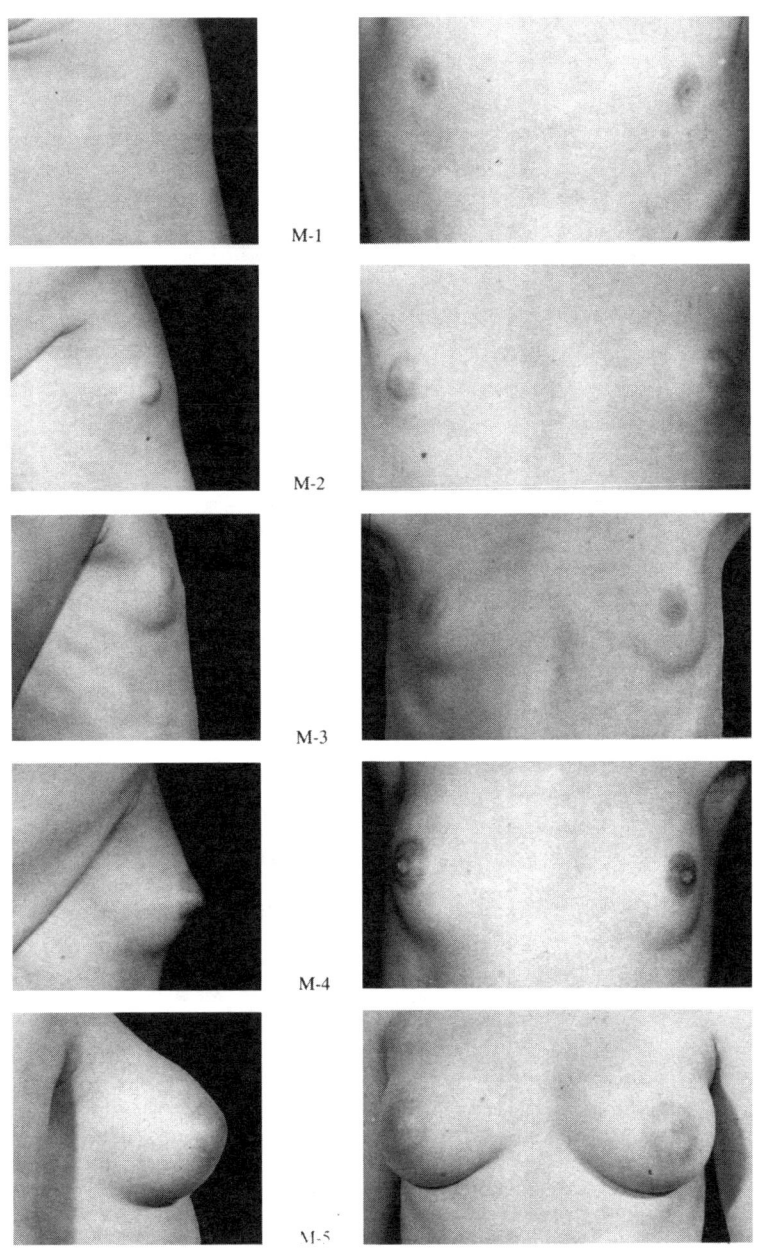

Fig 1. Stages of breast development in girls. M-1, Prepubertal, with no palpable breast tissue. M-2, Breast bud, elevation of the papilla and enlargement of the areolar diameter. M-3, Enlargement of the breast, without separation of the areolar contour from the breast. M-4, Formation of the secondary mound above the breast, from projection of the areola and papilla. M-5, Recession of the areola to the contour of the breast and the papilla beyond the contour of the areola and breast. (Reproduced from Roede MJ, van Wieringen JC. Growth diagrams 1980: Netherlands third nation-wide survey. *Tijdschr Soc Gezondheidsz.* 1985;63(suppl):1–34[no longer under copyright].)

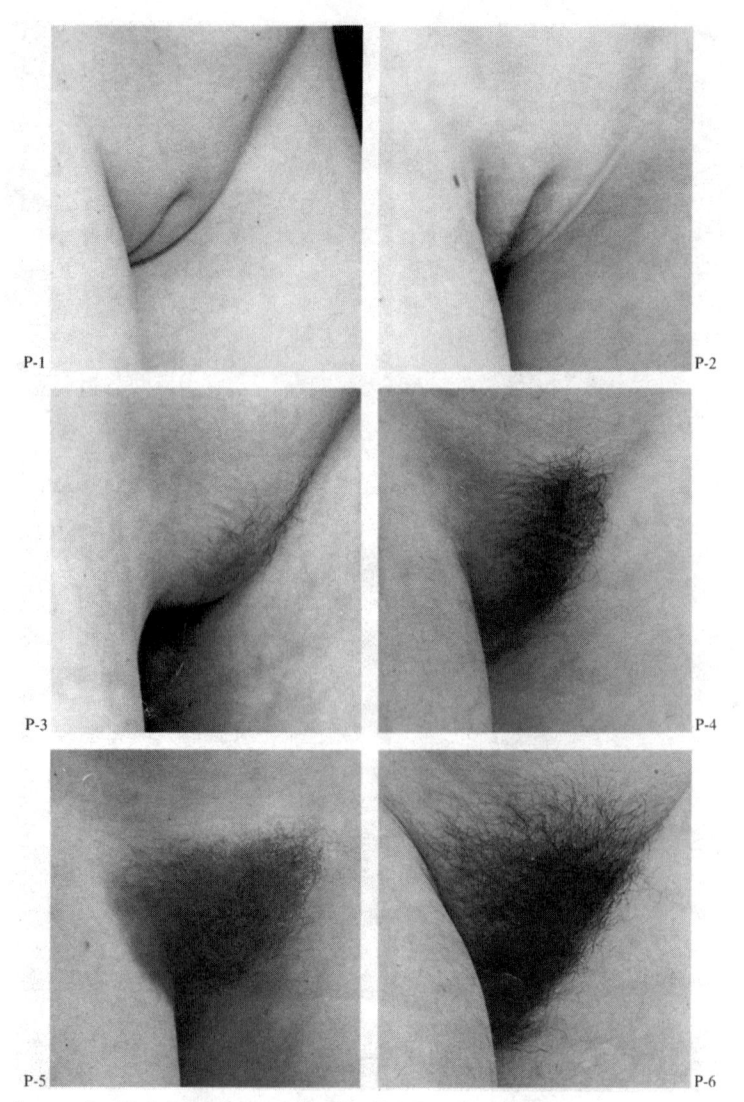

Fig 2. Stages of pubic hair development in girls. P-1, Prepubertal with no pubic hair. P-2, Sparse, straight hair along the lateral vulva. P-3, Hair is darker, coarser, and curlier, and extends over the midpubis. P-4, Hair is adult-like in appearance but does not extend to the thighs. P-5, Hair is adult in appearance and extends from thigh to thigh. (Reproduced from Roede MJ, van Wieringen JC. Growth diagrams 1980: Netherlands third nation-wide survey. *Tijdschr Soc Gezondheidsz.* 1985;63(suppl):1–34[no longer under copyright].)

precision of this staging system and prefer the measurement of testicular volume. In addition, measurement of testicular volume provides the clinician with important additional information.[7,8]

Figures 4 and 5 provide an opportunity to compare different biological events

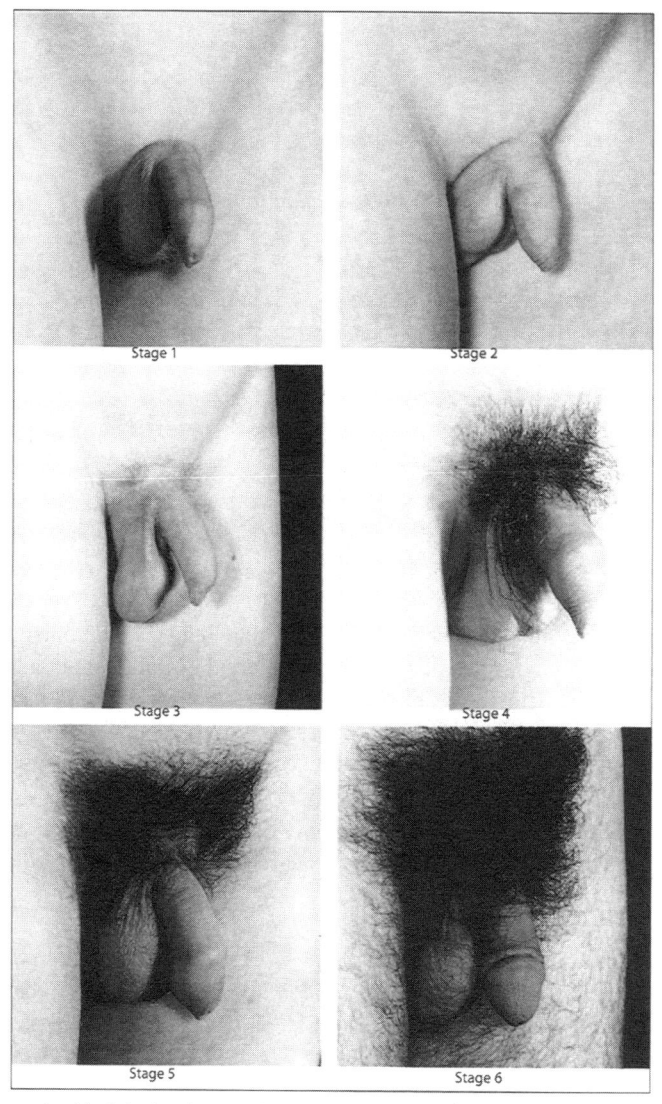

Fig 3 Stages of pubic hair development in boys. Stage 1, Prepubertal with no pubic hair. Stage 2, Sparse, straight hair along the base of the penis. Stage 3, Hair is darker, coarser, and curlier, and extends over the midpubis. Stage 4, Hair is adult-like in appearance but does not extend to the thighs. Stage 5, Hair is adult in appearance and extends from thigh to thigh. (Reproduced from Roede MJ, van Wieringen JC. Growth diagrams 1980: Netherlands third nation-wide survey. *Tijdschr Soc Gezondheidsz.* 1985;63(suppl):1–34[no longer under copyright].)

that occur during puberty in girls and boys, respectively. As shown in Fig 4, the earliest external sign of puberty in girls is an increase in growth velocity, which predates the appearance of secondary sexual characteristics. Most girls will have breast development before the appearance of pubic hair, and there is some

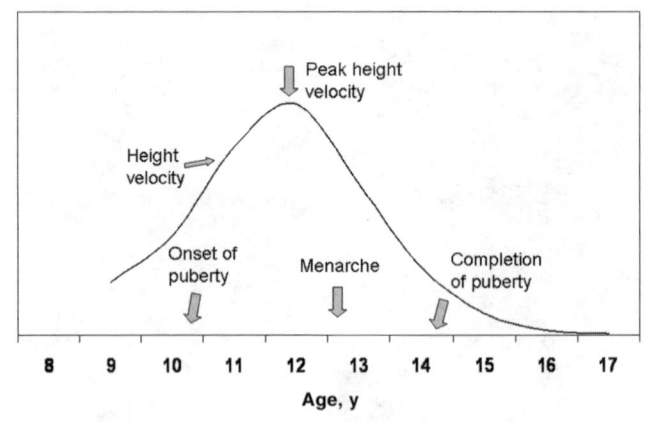

Fig 4. Sequence of pubertal events in girls. (Reproduced with permission from Biro FM, Huang B, Crawford PB, et al. Pubertal correlates in black and white girls. *J Pediatr.* 2006;148:234–240 and Biro FM. Puberty: whither goest? *J Pediatr Adolesc Gynecol.* 2006;19:163–165.)

controversy as to whether pubic hair development, without breast development, represents true puberty or isolated adrenarche. Returning to Fig 4, the peak height velocity in girls generally occurs before menarche, and the attainment of breast stage 5 and pubic hair stage 5 occurs shortly before the attainment of adult height. During puberty in girls, there are changes in body composition. A recent article noted that the change in BMI in girls up to age 16 typically leads to greater accrual of lean body mass rather than fat mass.[9]

In Fig 5, the earliest external change of pubertal maturation in boys is an increase in testicular volume, which is approximately concurrent with an increase in

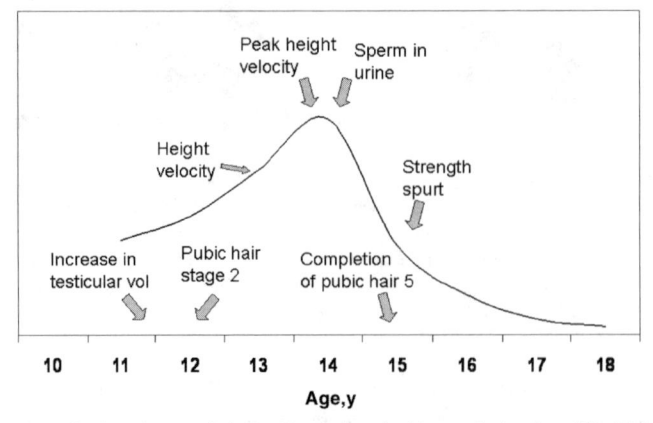

Fig 5. Sequence of pubertal events in boys. (Reproduced with permission from Biro FM. Adolescent medicine: requisites in pediatrics. In: Slap GB, ed. *Normal Growth and Development*. Philadelphia, PA: Elsevier; In press.)

growth velocity. Pubic hair develops ~6 to 9 months after the increase in testicular volume. Peak height velocity occurs around the same time as nocturnal emissions, as well as the appearance of sperm in the urine. Figure 5 also shows that growth continues in boys for 1 to 2 years after the attainment of pubic hair stage 5.

As most women will acknowledge, girls mature before boys, and males never quite catch up. Men are typically taller than women, partly because of differences in the timing of the growth spurt. Boys have an extra 1 to 2 years of slow prepubertal growth, they are generally 1 to 2 cm taller at 5 to 6 years of age, and peak height velocity is greater in boys than in girls.

Contemporary studies suggest that the age of onset of puberty may be occurring at younger ages than in the past, although the data are not entirely consistent. A study that compared several national studies (National Health Examination Survey and National Health and Nutrition Surveys) between 1996 and the later 1990s noted that there is a downward trend in the age of onset of puberty for white boys, as well as Hispanic boys and girls, but the data were not as conclusive for black boys or girls or white girls.[10]

From the perspective of any given adolescent, rather than national trends, for example, the timing of pubertal maturation affects final adult height and body composition, self-worth, risk-taking behaviors as an adolescent and an adult, and ultimate academic achievement. Girls who mature earlier are shorter and have a greater BMI.[11-14] Girls who mature earlier were noted to have poorer body image (although there was a significant interaction with BMI)[15] and more norm-breaking behaviors at ages 15 to 16.[16] As adults, girls who mature earlier had lower academic achievement[16] and higher rates of major depression and poorer relationships.[17] Boys who mature earlier or later had a greater risk of subclinical psychopathology,[17] and when late-maturing boys became adults, they were more likely to have current substance and/or tobacco abuse issues.[17]

COMMON MEDICAL ISSUES ASSOCIATED WITH PUBERTAL MATURATION

There are several common medical issues associated with pubertal maturation encountered by the clinician, including early or late timing, short stature, gynecomastia, acne, musculoskeletal problems, and myopia. Together, these have been termed the "perils of puberty."[18] The biological and social consequences of early maturation were discussed in the previous paragraph. The clinician will not encounter patients in their teenage years who present with early maturation because they would, by definition, mature earlier than their peers. The interested reader may wish to read several excellent reviews that have been published on the evaluation and management of those with early pubertal maturation.[19,20]

Late timing of pubertal maturation is identified by absent or incomplete development of the signs of puberty at a chronologic age by which 95% of the population would have begun puberty. Reviewing several recent publications, including the National Health and Nutrition Examination Survey and Pediatric Research in Office Settings,[21,22] ~95% of girls will begin puberty by age 12, and 95% of boys by age 13; traditionally, girls have begun puberty at 13 years of age and boys at 14 years of age. In a review of 232 adolescents referred for delayed puberty, boys outnumbered girls at a ratio of nearly 2:1, and the most common etiology was constitutional delay.[23] In constitutional delay, the bone age and height age are similar and are delayed when compared with chronologic age. In contrast, those with familial short stature will have a bone age consistent with chronologic age.

Gynecomastia is the development of breast tissue in a male. It occurs in the neonatal period, in old age, and in one half to two thirds of adolescent boys. Adolescent gynecomastia resolves spontaneously in nearly all cases within 18 to 24 months. If palpable tissue (as contrasted to adipose tissue in the chest) is >2 cm, or persists beyond 24 months, the adolescent should be evaluated for secondary causes such as Klinefelter syndrome, thyroid disease, or testicular tumors.

Acne occurs in essentially all male adolescents and most female adolescents. Girls with moderate-to-severe acne, irregular menses, evidence of excess androgens (such as clitoromegaly or excess body hair), and/or acanthosis nigricans may require evaluation for polycystic ovary syndrome, congenital adrenal hyperplasia, or insulin-resistant diabetes.

Musculoskeletal concerns during the adolescent period include sprains and strains, inflammation at sites of insertion of ligaments and tendons (apophysitis), stress fractures, epiphyseal instability, and scoliosis. The underlying mechanisms include rapid growth of linear height and weight and rapid bone turnover. In addition, teenaged girls encounter a rapid increase in the incidence of serious knee injuries, and this risk of injury persists into the adult years.[24]

Myopia begins or becomes worse during puberty. There are multiple factors, including increased near-vision activities during adolescence,[25] but there seem to be factors intrinsic to anatomic changes in the face, the ocular orbit, and globe that occur during the pubertal growth spurt.

CONCLUSIONS

Puberty is a time of profound biological changes that occur simultaneously with important cognitive and social change. There are several medical issues that arise or become more evident during puberty. Some changes are physiologic, whereas others are harbingers of more serious conditions.

REFERENCES

1. Hume D. *A Treatise of Human Nature.* Selby-Bigge LA, ed. London, England: Oxford University Press; 1896:415

2. Dahl RE. Adolescent brain development: a period of vulnerabilities and opportunities—keynote address. *Ann N Y Acad Sci.* 2004;1021:1–22
3. Giedd JN. Structural magnetic resonance imaging of the adolescent brain. *Ann N Y Acad Sci.* 2004;1021:77–85
4. Seminara SB, Messager S, Chatzidaki EE, et al. The GPR54 gene as a regulator of puberty. *N Engl J Med.* 2003;349:1614–1627
5. Tanner JM. *Growth at Adolescence.* 2nd ed. Oxford, United Kingdom: Blackwell Scientific; 1962
6. Roede MJ, van Wieringen JC. Growth diagrams 1980: Netherlands third nation-wide survey [in Dutch]. *Tijdschr Soc Gezondheidsz.* 1985;63(suppl):1–34
7. Biro FM, Lucky AW, Huster GA, Morrison JA. Pubertal staging in boys [published correction appears in *J Pediatr.* 1995;127:674]. *J Pediatr.* 1995;127:100–102
8. Largo RH, Prader A. Pubertal development in Swiss boys. *Helv Paediatr Acta.* 1983;38:211–228
9. Maynard LM, Wisemandle W, Roche AF, Chumlea WC, Guo SS, Siervogel RM. Childhood body composition in relation to body mass index. *Pediatrics.* 2001;107:344–350
10. Sun SS, Schubert CM, Liang R, et al. Is sexual maturity occurring earlier among U.S. children? *J Adolesc Health.* 2005;37:345–355
11. Biro FM, McMahon RP, Striegel-Moore R, et al. Impact of timing of pubertal maturation on growth in black and white female adolescents: the National Heart, Lung, and Blood Institute Growth and Health Study. *J Pediatr.* 2001;138:636–643
12. Freedman DS, Khan LK, Serdula MK, Dietz WH, Srinivasan SR, Berenson GS. Relation of age at menarche to race, time period, and anthropometric dimensions: the Bogalusa Heart Study. *Pediatrics.* 2002;110(4). Available at: www.pediatrics.org/cgi/content/full/110/4/e43
13. Kaplowitz PB, Slora EJ, Wasserman RC, Pedlow SE, Herman-Giddens ME. Earlier onset of puberty in girls: relation to increased body mass index and race. *Pediatrics.* 2001;108:347–353
14. Wang Y. Is obesity associated with early sexual maturation? A comparison of the association in American boys versus girls. *Pediatrics.* 2002;110:903–910
15. Striegel-Moore RH, McMahon RP, Biro FM, Schreiber G, Crawford PB, Voorhees C. Exploring the relationship between timing of menarche and eating disorder symptoms in black and white adolescent girls. *Int J Eat Disord.* 2001;30:421–433
16. Johansson T, Ritzen EM. Very long-term follow-up of girls with early and late menarche. *Endocr Dev.* 2005;8:126–136
17. Graber JA, Seeley JR, Brooks-Gunn J, Lewinsohn PM. Is pubertal timing associated with psychopathology in young adulthood? *J Am Acad Child Adolesc Psychiatry.* 2004;43:718–726
18. Biro F. Normal puberty. In: Rose BD, ed. UpToDate. Waltham, MA: UpToDate Press; 2007
19. Kaplowitz PB, Oberfield SE; Drug and Therapeutics and Executive Committees of the Lawson Wilkins Pediatric Endocrine Society. Reexamination of the age limit for defining when puberty is precocious in girls in the United States: implications for evaluation and treatment. *Pediatrics.* 1999;104:936–941
20. Muir A. Precocious puberty. *Pediatr Rev.* 2006;27:373–381
21. Herman-Giddens M, Slora E, Wasserman R, et al. Secondary sexual characteristics and menses in young girls seen in office practice: a study from the Pediatric Research in Office Settings network. *Pediatrics.* 1997;99:505–512
22. Sun SS, Schubert CM, Chumlea WC, et al. National estimates of the timing of sexual maturation and racial differences among US children. *Pediatrics.* 2002;110:911–919
23. Sedlmeyer IL, Palmert MR. Delayed puberty: analysis of a large case series from an academic center. *J Clin Endocrinol Metab.* 2002;87:1613–1620
24. Hewett TE, Lindenfeld TN, Riccobene JV, Noyes FR. The effect of neuromuscular training on the incidence of knee injury in female athletes: a prospective study. *Am J Sports Med.* 1999;27:699–706
25. Saw SM. A synopsis of the prevalence rates and environmental risk factors for myopia. *Clin Exp Optom.* 2003;86:289–294

Understanding Sexual Behaviors of Adolescents Within a Biopsychosocial Framework

Beth A. Auslander, PhD*[a], Susan L. Rosenthal, PhD[a], Margaret J. Blythe, MD[b]

[a]*Division of Adolescent and Behavioral Health, Department of Pediatrics and Sealy Center for Vaccine Development, University of Texas Medical Branch, 301 University Boulevard, Galveston, TX 77555-0319, USA*

[b]*Divisions of Adolescent Medicine and Community/General Pediatrics, Indiana University School of Medicine, 1001 West 10th Street, Bryce Building, Room B2006, Indianapolis, IN 46202, USA*

Adolescent sexual behavior is best understood within a biopsychosocial framework. In this article, we first discuss how pubertal development and social influences come together to shape adolescent sexual behaviors. We then present data on noncoital and coital behaviors among adolescent populations and pay special attention to variations across gender and race/ethnicities. We conclude with a review of the data on teen pregnancy and sexually transmitted infection (STI) rates within the United States.

Typically, adolescence is the period between 10 and 20 years of age, and it often is divided into 3 phases, including early (10- to 14-year-olds), middle (15- to 17-year-olds), and late (18- to 20-year-olds). During adolescence, individuals experience pubertal changes, begin to develop higher-level cognitive skills, start the separation-individuation process wherein they begin to move away from parents and develop closer attachments with peers and romantic partners, and begin to experience sexual feelings and attractions. These changes take place in a social context that may influence their expression. For example, studies indicate that the earlier pubertal development occurs, the more susceptible an adolescent is to initiate sexual behavior and to have a greater number of sexual experiences.[1-4] However, earlier maturation does not result in the earlier development of higher-level cognitive reasoning (eg, abstract reasoning), thus poten-

---

*Corresponding author.
E-mail address: baasulan@utmb.edu (B. A. Auslander).

Copyright © 2007 American Academy of Pediatrics. All rights reserved. ISSN 1934-4287

tially placing early maturers at more risk for making unhealthy sexual decisions than their same-aged peers with no pubertal changes. In addition to the developmental differences that occur with age that may place them at risk sexually, adolescents who are the same age may have individual differences that place them at risk sexually. Higher levels of testosterone are associated with a greater likelihood of initiating sexual behavior and having more sexual experiences among both males and females.[1,2] Those who have lower overall cognitive abilities and/or less confidence in specific problem-solving skills often required for the negotiation of abstinence and the use of condoms are thus more likely to engage in sex[5] and less likely to use condoms consistently.[6]

Because these developmental and individual differences exist in a social context, risk can be mediated. For example, research has documented that when parents monitor their adolescents closely and communicate their disapproval about having sex at an early age, adolescents are more likely to delay sexual activity and use protection.[7-10] Peers also play a role. Adolescents who perceive that their peers recognize the benefits of abstinence and who believe that few of their peers are sexually active are less likely to have initiated intercourse.[11,12] Higher levels of religiosity and higher socioeconomic status have been linked to a later age of sexual initiation.[11] Thus, although an individual may be prone to initiate sexual intercourse at a young age as a result of early pubertal development, certain social influences can provide a protective role and help delay the onset of sexual behavior. Parental influences and religiosity and spirituality as factors that influence adolescent sexuality are discussed more in depth by Rupp and Rosenthal[13] and Cotton and Berry,[14] respectively, later in this issue.

ADOLESCENT SEXUAL BEHAVIORS

Most adolescents have had some form of sexual contact, with 75% of them having engaged in deep kissing by the end of high school.[15] A landmark study published in 1985[16] revealed that, at least for white adolescents, a gradual unfolding pattern of sexual behavior emerges, wherein individuals first engage in kissing, then breast touching, then genital touching, and finally sexual intercourse. It is interesting to note that this predictable pattern was not present among black adolescents, which suggests that 1 pattern does not fit adolescents of all backgrounds and cultures. Only recently have oral and anal sex been thoroughly studied; thus, it is not clear how they fit within the above-mentioned pattern. Understanding how the variety of sexual behaviors fit within adolescent lives will help health care providers to counsel adolescents about sexual decision-making behaviors and STI risk.

Masturbation

Masturbation is defined as self-stimulation of the genitals for the purpose of sexual arousal, not necessarily leading to orgasm.[17] Attitudes toward the role of masturbation in one's sexual life vary. Some people view masturbation negatively (eg, masturbation is sinful because it prevents procreation), others more neutrally (eg, it is a normal behavior in a person's developing sexuality that is good unless used in excess), and still others more positively (eg, masturbation is a healthy sexual behavior that allows one to explore his or her sexuality and experience pleasure).[17] There is no evidence that masturbation during adolescence is either harmful or beneficial to one's sexual development or later adult sexual adjustment. Masturbation during early adolescence is not related to early sexual intercourse,[18] sexual satisfaction, sexual arousal, or sexual problems within a relationship.[19]

The first studies on masturbation were conducted by Kinsey[20,21] in the 1940s and 1950s and revealed that more males than females had engaged in it. This gender difference in masturbatory practices has been found to be present as early as preadolescence and population samples from Sweden, Australia, and the United States.[18,19,22] The biggest gender difference was found among college students in the northeastern United States: 81% of the males and 45% of the females had ever masturbated.[19] Gender differences also exist with respect to frequency of masturbation. In a report by Leitenberg et al,[19] males reported a masturbatory frequency during adolescence and young adulthood that was 3 times that of females. It is interesting to note that there are no differences across gender in the age of initiation of masturbation. Both males and females report first masturbating between 12 and 14 years of age, with most reporting that they learned to masturbate through self-discovery.[18]

Researchers have postulated that biological factors, such as hormones and arousal stimulated by friction of the penis against clothing, are in part responsible for the gender differences in masturbation practices.[19] Sociocultural factors also have been suggested to explain the differences. Although masturbation is an expected behavior for males in Western cultures, it still may be considered taboo for females. Girls are expected to associate sexual behavior with emotional connection or intimacy rather than engage in it for purely sexual or physical reasons.[19] A study revealed that parents communicate different expectations or attitudes toward masturbation that are based on the gender of their child.[23] When parents found their sons masturbating, they often instructed their sons to go somewhere private to engage in this behavior, whereas when parents found their daughters masturbating, they often lectured the daughters about the inappropriateness and immorality of the behavior.[23] Given the societal messages to girls regarding masturbation, it is not surprising that many young college women experience guilt associated with masturbatory practices.[24]

A few studies have investigated adolescents' experience with "masturbation of" or "by a partner," sometimes also referred to as "mutual masturbation without penetrative sex" or "outercourse."[25,26] More adolescents have participated in this behavior than sexual intercourse, as evidenced by the fact that both "virgins" (ie, those who have not had vaginal intercourse) and "nonvirgins" (ie, those who have had vaginal intercourse) have engaged in this behavior. The prevalence rates range from 16% to 29% among virgins who have ever masturbated a partner and from 16% to 31% for those who have ever been masturbated by a partner.[26–28] Among a US sample of 17- to 19-year-old heterosexual nonvirgin males, 78% reported having masturbated a partner or been masturbated by a partner.[27] These percentages did not differ significantly by gender but did differ with regard to race/ethnicity, with Asian and Pacific Islander adolescents being less likely than white, black, and Latino adolescents to have masturbated by themselves or with a partner.[28] Some educators of STI/HIV-prevention programs encourage the inclusion of mutual masturbation/outercourse as a safer-sex behavior along with abstinence and consistent condom use. One program that provided education about these 3 safe-sex behaviors was found to increase HIV-positive youths' use of outercourse and safer-sex behaviors as a whole.[29]

Oral Sex

Descriptions of the prevalence rates of oral sex among adolescents vary across studies on the basis of the definition used in the study, which included the following: "fellatio," "fellatio with ejaculation," "cunnilingus," "receptive oral sex," "received oral sex," "gave oral sex," and simply "oral sex."[26–28,30,31]

How adolescents view oral sex and reasons for engaging in it are complex. Sixty percent of undergraduates reported that they did not consider themselves to have "had sex" if they had engaged in oral sex only.[32] Researchers have suggested that adolescents substitute oral sex for vaginal sex to retain their virginity status.[28,32–34] It is clear that adolescent virgins (ie, those who have not experienced vaginal intercourse) engage in oral sex. Studies have indicated prevalence rates that range from 4% to 35%.[26,27,33,35,36] Approximately 57% to 70% of adolescents indicated that they engaged in oral sex before the onset of vaginal intercourse.[37,38] Previous research has also indicated that some adolescents prefer oral sex over vaginal sex because it allows them to experience sexual pleasure while at the same time they can avoid the social, emotional, and physical health risks associated with vaginal sex.[39–41] That is, adolescents who have engaged in oral sex behaviors only, compared with those who have engaged in both oral and vaginal sexual behaviors, are less likely to report having had an STI or pregnancy, to have felt guilty, to have gotten in trouble with their parents, and to have experienced problems in their romantic relationships.[41] Among nonvirgins, oral sex serves as another form of sexual expression, and prevalence rates suggest that from 63% to 84%[27,28,35,42] have engaged in oral sex at some point.

Attitudes toward oral sex seem to be culturally derived, as seen in the differences in attitudes between males and females and the differences in prevalence and attitudes across racial/ethnic groups. Although it seems that males and females engage in oral sex at similar rates,[30,38,39,43] the behavior is viewed differently across genders. Males have been shown to have more accepting attitudes, and greater numbers of males expect to be given oral sex than females.[37,44] Males and females seem to engage in oral sex for different reasons, with adolescent girls more likely than adolescent boys to state the following reasons for why teenagers have oral sex: personal benefits, social factors, fear, control, and improvement of the romantic relationship.[40]

Oral sex also has been found to be less prevalent among Asian and Pacific Islander adolescents than it is among white, black, and Latino adolescents[28] and less prevalent among black men and women than white men and women.[45] Generally, although black women initiate sexual intercourse at an earlier age than white women, black women initiate oral sex at a later age than white women.[45] However, the gap in oral sex rates between blacks and whites seems to be getting smaller, with increasing prevalence rates among blacks and stable rates among whites and Hispanics.[27]

To our knowledge, 3 studies have examined parental influence on adolescent oral sexual behaviors. It seems that few parents have conversations with their adolescents about oral sex (16% of young adult females).[33] It is unclear if having a conversation provides any protective benefit.[46] In general, adolescents think that they will get in less trouble with their parents for having oral sex than vaginal sex.[41] Whether they believe they would have less consequences, because they actually would get in less trouble or because there has been no conversation about the subject of oral sex is unknown.

Peers seem to play a role in adolescent oral sex behaviors. Adolescents who perceive their peers to approve of oral sex or to have had oral sex are more likely to have had oral sex themselves.[30,46] Also, a positive correlation between the number of an adolescent's oral-sex partners and his or her perceived number of friends' oral-sex partners has been found.[30] From the peer perspective, adolescents who have had oral sex are rated more highly on popularity measures.[30] Thus, it could be that sexually active adolescents are more popular than their nonsexually active peers, or perhaps popular adolescents are more likely to report being sexually active. These findings underscore the importance of addressing peer influences when counseling peers on the subject of oral-sex behaviors.

STIs are more easily spread through vaginal or anal intercourse than oral sex. However, several STIs, including gonorrhea and syphilis, and viral STIs, such as herpes simplex virus types 1 and 2 (HSV-1 and HSV-2) and HIV, can be transmitted through oral sex.[47,48] The per-contact risk of acquiring HIV through receptive oral intercourse with a known HIV-positive or unknown serostatus partner has been estimated at 0.04%.[49] It has been suggested that 6% to 8% of new HIV infections result from unprotected oral intercourse.[50] Recent studies have suggested that more and more genital herpes cases are caused by HSV-1, suggesting oral sex as the mode of transmission.[31] In a recent study, ~2% of the adolescents who experienced oral sex only (ie, no history of vaginal intercourse) reported that they acquired an STI.[41]

Adolescents seem aware that health risks associated with oral sex are much lower than those associated with vaginal intercourse.[39] However, of concern is that ~13% to 32% of adolescents do not perceive any risk of acquiring STIs/HIV from oral sex.[37,39,43] In addition, previous research has suggested that most adolescents typically do not use protection during oral sex.[37,43] Given these findings, it seems important for health care providers to be aware of and educate adolescents about the risks associated with oral sex.

Anal Intercourse

Although a relatively uncommon adolescent behavior (prevalence rates range from 1% to 32%),[26,51] anal intercourse is still an important sexual behavior of adolescents given the risk of transmission and acquisition of STIs, including HIV, and the association of anal intercourse with other risk-taking behaviors. Unfortunately, it is rarely studied, and discussions of anal intercourse are often considered taboo.[51,52]

Prevalence of anal intercourse seems to vary across adolescent populations on the basis of virginity status and age. Among a sample of so-called virgin male and female adolescents in grades 9 through 12, 1% had engaged in anal intercourse.[26] In a sample of 15- to 19-year-old heterosexual males, some of whom were virgins and some of whom were nonvirgins, 11% reported having had anal intercourse.[27] Among college populations, the prevalence rates of anal intercourse increases somewhat, ranging from 17% to 32%.[51-54] The average age of initiation of anal intercourse is between 18 and 20 years,[52-54] with males initiating anal intercourse at a younger age than females.[54] Heterosexual males also have been found to engage in anal intercourse more frequently than females.[54]

Adolescents and college students who have had anal intercourse tend to make more risky sexual decisions than those who have not. Studies show that compared with those who have not had anal intercourse, those with such experience began having vaginal intercourse at a younger age,[51,52,55] have had more lifetime sexual partners,[51,53] and are less likely to have reported using condoms during their last vaginal intercourse.[52] Although anal intercourse carries a higher risk of transmission of HIV and other STIs than vaginal intercourse, adolescents and college students do not seem to be paying attention to this risk. Among a college sample of males and females, condoms were used only 21% of the time during anal intercourse versus 43% of the time during vaginal intercourse in the 3 months before data collection.[52] It is not surprising that the reported STI rates are higher among those with a history of anal sex.[51]

Vaginal Sexual Intercourse

A 2005 survey of US high school students (Youth Risk Behavior Surveillance Survey [YRBSS]) and the 2002 National Survey of Family Growth of 15- to 19-year old never-married adolescents indicated that ~46% to 47% of those in this group have engaged in sexual intercourse.[56,57] On a positive note, analysis of the YRBSS from 1991 to 2005 and a comparison of the 1995 and 2002 National Surveys of Family Growth indicate that the prevalence rates of ever having engaged in intercourse, of having multiple sex partners, and of currently being sexual active have decreased, whereas condom use and other types of contraceptive use, including use of both barrier and hormonal methods, increased among adolescents.[56,58] As can be seen in Fig 1, the prevalence rates for sexual behaviors have steadily leveled off since 2001.[58]

Experience with vaginal sexual intercourse seems to be developmentally and culturally driven, because there are variations in prevalence rates for sex by age and race/ethnicity, in partner accrual by age, gender, and race/ethnicity, in age of sexual initiation by gender and race/ethnicity, and in condom use by gender and race/ethnicity. For instance, on the 2005 YRBSS,[57] more students in grades 10 through 12 had engaged in vaginal intercourse than students in grade 9, and the prevalence rates of vaginal intercourse were higher among black and Hispanic students than among white students. Higher percentages of older students than younger students, males than females, and black students than white and Hispanic students have had 4 or more lifetime sexual partners. More males than females and more black students than white and Hispanic students have had sex before they were 13 years old. With regard to condom use at last intercourse, the prevalence rates were higher among males than females and among black students than white and Hispanic students.[57]

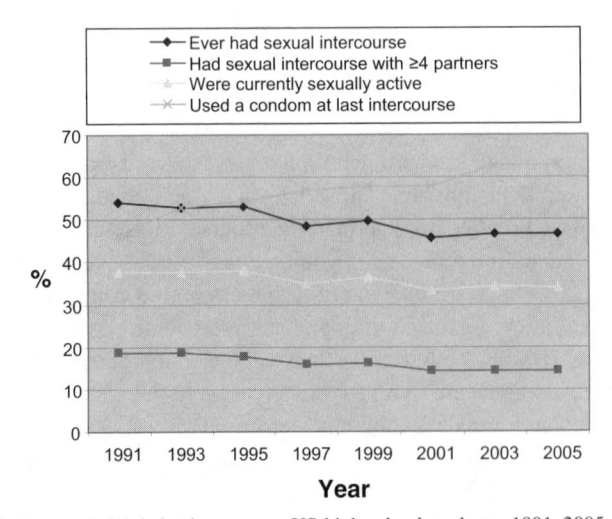

Fig 1. Trends in sexual risk behaviors among US high school students: 1991–2005.

Given the costs associated with early sexual initiation and unprotected sex, researchers have attempted to identify social factors associated with delay in sexual activity and safe-sex behaviors. A recent review of studies[59] that examined predictors of adolescent sexual behavior indicated that adolescents whose parents disapprove of their having sex are more likely than adolescents without this characteristic to be abstinent and to engage in less risky sexual behaviors. This same review indicated that the findings with regard to the relationship between parental monitoring and adolescent sexual behavior have been inconsistent, possibly because of methodologic reasons. Although 13 studies found that parental monitoring was associated with better sexual decisions among adolescents, 10 studies found no relationship between parental monitoring and adolescent sexual behavior. This review[59] also indicated that peer sex behaviors and attitudes toward sex were strong predictors of adolescent sexual behavior. When adolescents perceive that their peers have not had sex or believe that their peers have less favorable attitudes toward sex or early childbearing, they are more likely to make healthy sexual decisions such as delaying sexual behavior. Connection with community agencies such as school or church also seems to have a protective effect on adolescent sexual behavior.[11,60,61] Rupp and Rosenthal[13] present more discussion about parental influences in this issue.

Focusing on reasons or factors associated with delaying sexual activity or engaging in safe-sex behaviors yields valuable necessary information but is only 1 piece of the puzzle. It does not tell us why adolescents have sex and why they have unprotected sex. A recent study found that young adolescents expect that sexual intercourse will lead to improved intimacy, sexual pleasure, and higher social status for them.[62] Adolescents' perceptions of the benefits of sex and unprotected sex seem to differ by gender, sexual experience, and type of sexual relationship.[62,63] In 1 study, females viewed intimacy and social status as more important motivations to have sex than did males.[62] Younger and less sexually experienced adolescents perceive social status/peer influence as a major reason to have sex, whereas older adolescents report that they engage in sexual intercourse because they were in love, felt romantic, were physically attracted to their partner, felt too exited to stop, or had a partner who was drunk or high.[62,64] Of importance is that the perceived benefits of unprotected sex were found to be better predictors of sexual risk behaviors among adolescents than the perceived benefits and costs of using condoms.[65] Thus, it is critical that STI/HIV-prevention programs not only address the risks associated with adolescent sex-taking but also address the perceived benefits of both protected and unprotected sex. For example, because adolescents expect that sexual intercourse will lead to greater intimacy in their relationship, it would be helpful for STI/HIV-prevention programs to educate adolescents about the meaning of intimacy and provide ways other than vaginal intercourse to achieve intimacy within a romantic relationship.

NEGATIVE CONSEQUENCES OF ADOLESCENT SEXUAL BEHAVIOR

Pregnancy/Birth Rates

According to recent surveys, ~750 000 adolescents in the United States experience a pregnancy each year.[66] The number of teen pregnancies decreased by 27% from 1990 to 2000.[67] In 2005, among unmarried females from 10 to 19 years old, there were an estimated 421 000 births, with 20% being a second or later birth.[68] The birth rate for 15- to 19-year-old adolescents was 40.4 births per 1000 and was higher among Hispanic (81.5) and black youth (61) than white youth (26). Since 1991, the teenage birth rate has declined 45% and is at its lowest rate since the inception of a rating system by the National Center for Health Statistics.[68] Decreases in birth rates are more notable among 15- to 17-year-olds and among black youth.[68] Abortion rates among 10- to 19-year-old adolescents also seem to have been on the decline, decreasing 39% from the mid- to late 1980s to the year 2002.[69] Reasons for declines in teenage pregnancies and births are thought to be mostly a result of the increase in condom use and more reliable methods of birth control, as well as the decrease in numbers of adolescents initiating sexual intercourse.[56,70,71]

Most adolescents do not have favorable attitudes about the idea of becoming pregnant as a teen.[72] Although most teenage pregnancies are not intended, data from the National Longitudinal Study of Adolescent Health indicate that 14% of 15- to 19-year-old female adolescents reported feeling ambivalent toward becoming pregnant, and 8% reported having positive attitudes toward pregnancy.[73] The percentage of those with favorable attitudes toward pregnancy increased to 34% among those experiencing a "rapid-repeat" second pregnancy (defined as a pregnancy within 24 months of giving birth).[74] Favorable attitudes toward pregnancy also vary across cultures with Hispanic female adolescents perceiving more positive consequences from childbearing than other races/ethnicities. Understanding adolescents' perceptions toward pregnancy is important, because it predicts pregnancy risk. Adolescents who are ambivalent about becoming pregnant and those who perceive more positive consequences associated with having a child have been found to use contraceptives less consistently and are more likely to become pregnant than adolescents who have unfavorable views of pregnancy.[72,73,75]

Adolescent pregnancy is associated with negative consequences for both the mother and the infant. Compared with older mothers, teen mothers are less likely to achieve educational goals and to participate in the labor force and are more prone to poverty,[76,77] STDs,[78] and depression.[79] For infants, major complications, including death, prematurity, and low birth weight, are more prevalent among infants of teenaged mothers than infants of older mothers.[80,81] In addition, children of teenaged mothers are more likely than children of older mothers to experience health, cognitive, emotional, and behavioral problems.[82]

STIs

STIs continue to be a public health problem for adolescents. This age group is especially vulnerable to contracting STIs for biological reasons such as an underdeveloped cervix and immature immune system,[83,84] for behavioral reasons such as unprotected intercourse, and due to potential barriers to accessing health care.[85]

It is alarming that of the estimated 18.9 million new STI infections each year, 9.1 million occur in the 15- to 24-year-old age group.[86] Compared with the other age groups and with males, the highest rates of chlamydia and gonorrhea in the United States are among 15- to 19-year-old females at 2796 per 100 000 and 624.9 per 100 000, respectively.[87] Adolescents are also at a high risk for viral STIs. Human papillomavirus infections are the most common STIs among adolescents in the United States[86] and have prevalence rates of 24.5% among 14- to 19-year-old US females.[88] Genital herpes can result from HSV-1 infection, or more commonly, HSV-2 infection. A recent review of studies on the seroprevalence of HSV-1 and HSV-2 among adolescents in the United States indicated that ~53% of adolescent males and 49% of adolescent females are infected with HSV-1 and 12% of adolescent males and 15% of adolescent females are infected with HSV-2.[89] On a positive note, data from national surveys suggest that the seroprevalance of HSV-2 among US adolescents declined between 1988 and 2004.[90] In 2005, there were an estimated 1225 newly diagnosed cases of HIV/AIDS among 15- to 19-year-old adolescents reported in 33 US states and dependent territories, which is a 21% increase for this age group from 2001.[91]

STIs can cause serious and long-term health problems for adolescents, including pelvic inflammatory disease, infertility, pregnancy complications, and cervical cancer.[92,93] Their children can also suffer significant consequences (by means of vertical transmission) such as blindness, neurologic complications, and possibly death.[94-96] Unfortunately, HSV infections are lifelong infections and can also place a person at increased risk for transmitting and acquiring HIV/AIDS.[97] Adolescents diagnosed with an STI can also suffer psychological consequences, such as depression,[98] and they may engage more in self-blame and less in effective problem solving.[99]

CONCLUSIONS

Adolescence is a period of marked developmental changes during which individuals begin to experience sexual feelings and to engage in sexual behaviors that may place them at risk for unwanted pregnancy and STIs. When counseling adolescents about healthy sexual decision-making, health care providers should be aware of adolescent development and the psychosocial influences on sexual behavior, as well as the prevalence associated with a variety of adolescent behaviors. The decreases in adolescent sexual behaviors, increases in use of STI protection, and declining rates of teen pregnancy and births suggest that we as parents, communities, and health care providers are making a difference in adolescent sexual decisions. To forge ahead, we must continue to strive to understand sexual behavior from the adolescent viewpoint and within the adolescent social context. This will require that we begin to ask questions not only about vaginal sex but also about other types of sexual behaviors, that we further our knowledge about sociocultural factors that mediate the relationship between biological factors and sexual behavior, and that we acknowledge that adolescents perceive there to be benefits of sexual behaviors that at times for them may outweigh the costs. With such knowledge, we will be much better equipped to design effective interventions that prevent teen pregnancy and STIs and promote the sexual health of adolescents.

REFERENCES

1. Halpern CT, Udry JR, Suchindran C. Testosterone predicts initiation of coitus in adolescent females. *Psychosom Med.* 1997;59:161–171
2. Halpern CT, Udry JR, Suchindran C. Monthly measure of salivary testosterone predict sexual activity in adolescent males. *Arch Sex Behav.* 1998;27:445–465
3. Lam TH, Shi HJ, Ho LM, Stewart SM, Fan S. Timing of pubertal maturation and heterosexual behavior among Hong Kong Chinese Adolescents. *Arch Sex Behav.* 2002;31:359–366
4. Ostovich JM, Sabini J. Timing of puberty and sexuality in men and women. *Arch Sex Behav.* 2005;34:197–206
5. Halpern CT, Joyner K, Udry R, Suchindran C. Smart teens don't have sex (or kiss much either). *J Adolesc Health.* 2000;26:213–225
6. DiIorio C, Dudley WN, Kelly M, Soet JE, Mbwara J, Sharpe Potter J. Social cognitive correlates of sexual experience and condom use among 13- through 15-year-old adolescents. *J Adolesc Health.* 2001;29:208–216
7. Murry VM. Black adolescent females: a comparison of early versus late coital initiators. *Fam Relat.* 1994;43:342–348
8. Sieving RE, McNeely CS, Blum RW. Maternal expectations, mother-child connectedness, and adolescent sexual debut. *Arch Pediatr Adolesc Med.* 2000;154:809–816
9. McNeely C, Shew ML, Beuhring T, Sieving R, Miller BC, Blum RW. Mothers' influence on the timing of first sex among 14- and 15-year-olds. *J Adolesc Health.* 2002;31:256–265
10. Meschke LL, Silbereisen RK. The influence of puberty, family processes, and leisure activities on the timing of first sexual experience. *J Adolesc.* 1997;20:403–418
11. Lammers C, Ireland M, Resnick M, Blum R. Influences on adolescents' decision to postpone onset of sexual intercourse: a survival analysis of virginity among youths aged 13 to 18 years. *J Adolesc Health.* 2000;26:42–48
12. L'Engle KL, Jackson C, Brown JD. Early adolescents' cognitive susceptibility to initiating sexual intercourse. *Perspect Sex Reprod Health.* 2006;38:97–105
13. Rupp R, Rosenthal S. Parental influences on adolescent sexual behaviors. *Adolesc Med.* 2007;18:460–470
14. Cotton S, Berry D. Religiosity, spirituality, and adolescent sexuality. *Adolesc Med.* 2007;18:471–483
15. Roper Starch Worldwide Inc. *Teens Talk About Sex: Adolescent Sexuality in the 90's—A Survey of High School Students.* New York, NY: SIECUS; 1994

16. Smith EA, Udry JR. Coital and non-coital sexual behaviors of white and black adolescents. *Am J Public Health*. 1985;75:1200–1203
17. Sparrow M. Masturbation and safer sex: clinical, historical, and social issues. *Venereology*. 1994;7:164–169
18. Smith AM, Rosenthal DA, Reichler H. High schoolers' masturbatory practices: their relationship to sexual intercourse and personal characteristics. *Psychol Rep*. 1996;79:499–509
19. Leitenberg H, Detzer MJ, Srebnik D. Gender differences in masturbation and the relation of masturbation experience in preadolescence and/or early adolescence to sexual behavior and sexual adjustment in young adulthood. *Arch Sex Behav*. 1993;22:87–98
20. Kinsey AC, Pomeroy WB, Martin C, Gebhard, PH. *Sexual Behavior in the Human Female*. Philadelphia, PA: WB Saunders; 1953
21. Kinsey AC, Pomeroy WB, Martin CE. *Sexual Behavior in the Human Male*. Philadelphia, PA: WB Saunders; 1948
22. Larsson I, Svedin CG. Sexual experiences in childhood: young adults' recollections. *Arch Sex Behav*. 2002;31:263–273
23. Gagnon JH. Attitudes and responses of parents to pre-adolescent masturbation. *Arch Sex Behav*. 1985;14:451–466
24. Davidson JK, Moore NB. Masturbation and premarital sexual intercourse among college women: making choices for sexual fulfillment. *J Sex Marital Ther*. 1994;20:178–199
25. Ehrhardt AA. Our view of adolescent sexuality: a focus on risk behavior without the developmental context. *Am J Public Health*. 1996;86:1523–1525
26. Schuster MA, Bell RM, Kanouse DE. The sexual practices of adolescent virgins: genital sexual activities of high school students who have never had vaginal intercourse. *Am J Public Health*. 1996;86:1570–1576
27. Gates GJ, Sonenstein FL. Heterosexual genital sexual activity among adolescent males: 1988 and 1995. *Fam Plann Perspect*. 2000;32:295–297, 304
28. Schuster MA, Bell RM, Nakajima GA, Kanouse DE. The sexual practices of Asian and Pacific Islander high school students. *J Adolesc Health*. 1998;23:221–231
29. Butler RB, Schultz JR, Forsberg AD, et al. Promoting safer sex among HIV-positive youth with haemophilia: theory, intervention, and outcome. *Haemophilia*. 2003;9:214–222
30. Prinstein MJ, Meade C, Cohen G. Adolescent oral sex, peer popularity, and perceptions of best friends' sexual behavior. *J Pediatr Psychol*. 2003;28:243–249
31. Lafferty WE, Downey L, Celum C, Wald A. Herpes simplex virus type I as a cause of genital herpes: impact on surveillance and prevention. *J Infect Dis*. 2000;181:1454–1457
32. Sanders SA, Reinisch JM. Would you say you "had sex" if . . .? *JAMA*. 1999;281:275–277
33. Herold ES, Way L. Oral-genital sexual behavior in a sample of university females. *J Sex Res*. 1983;19:327–338
34. Remez L. Oral sex among adolescents: is it sex or is it abstinence? *Fam Plann Perspect*. 2000;32:298–304
35. Newcomer S, Udry JR. Oral sex in an adolescent population. *Arch Sex Behav*. 1985;14:41–46
36. Mosher WD, Chandra A, Jones A. Sexual behavior and selected health measures: men and women 15–44 years of age, United States, 2002. *Adv Data*. 2005;(362):1–55
37. Stone N, Hatherall B, Ingham R, McEachran J. Oral sex and condom use among young people in the United Kingdom. *Perspect Sex Reprod Health*. 2006;38:6–12
38. Schwartz IM. Sexual activity prior to coital initiation: a comparison between males and females. *Arch Sex Behav*. 1999;28:63–69
39. Halpern-Felsher BL, Cornell JL, Kropp RY, Tschann JM. Oral versus vaginal sex among adolescents: perceptions, attitudes, and behavior. *Pediatrics*. 2005;115:845–851
40. Cornell JL, Halpern-Felsher BL. Adolescents tell us why teens have oral sex. *J Adolesc Health*. 2006;38:299–301
41. Brady SS, Halpern-Felsher BL. Adolescents' reported consequences of having oral sex versus vaginal sex. *Pediatrics*. 2007;119:229–236

42. Feldman L, Holowaty P, Harvey B, Rannie K, Shortt L, Jamal A. A comparison of the demographic, lifestyle, and sexual behaviour characteristics of virgin and non-virgin adolescents. *Can J Hum Sex*. 1997;6:197–209
43. Boekeloo BO, Howard DE. Oral sexual experience among young adolescents receiving general health examinations. *Am J Health Behav*. 2002;26:306–314
44. Wilson SM, Medora NP. Gender comparisons of college students' attitudes toward sexual behavior. *Adolescence*. 1990;25:615–627
45. Ompad DC, Strathdee SA, Celentano DD, et al. Predictors of early initiation of vaginal and oral sex among urban young adults in Baltimore, Maryland. *Arch Sex Behav*. 2006;35:53–65
46. Bersamin MM, Walker S, Fisher DA, Grube JW. Correlates of oral sex and vaginal intercourse in early and middle adolescence. *J Res Adolesc*. 2006;16:59–68
47. Edwards S, Carne C. Oral sex and transmission of non-viral STIs. *Sex Transm Infect*. 1998;74:95–100
48. Edwards S, Carne C. Oral sex and the transmission of viral STIs. *Sex Transm Infect*. 1998;74:6–10
49. Vittinghoff E, Douglas J, Judson F, McKirnan D, MacQueen K, Buchbinder SP. Per-contact risk of human immunodeficiency virus transmission between male sexual partners. *Am J Epidemiol*. 1999;150:306–311
50. Hawkins D. Oral sex and HIV transmission. *Sex Transm Infect*. 2001;77:307–308
51. Flannery D, Ellingson L, Votaw KS, Schaefer EA. Anal intercourse and sexual risk factors among college women: 1993–2000. *Am J Health Behav*. 2003;27:228–234
52. Baldwin JI, Baldwin JD. Heterosexual anal intercourse: an understudied, high-risk sexual behavior. *Arch Sex Behav*. 2000;29:357–373
53. Reinisch JM, Sanders SA, Hill CA, Ziemba-Davis M. High-risk sexual behavior among heterosexual undergraduates at a midwestern university. *Fam Plann Perspect*. 1992;24:116–121, 145
54. Reinisch JM, Hill CA, Sanders SA, Ziemba-Davis M. High-risk sexual behavior at a midwestern university: a confirmatory survey. *Fam Plann Perspect*. 1995;27:79–82
55. Edgardh K. Sexual behaviour and early coitarche in a national sample of 17-year-old Swedish girls. *Sex Transm Infect*. 2000;76:98–102
56. Abma J, Martinez GM, Mosher WD, Dawson B. Teenagers in the United States: sexual activity, contraceptive use, and childbearing, 2002. *Vital Health Stat 23*. 2004;(24):1–48
57. Centers for Disease Control and Prevention. Youth Risk Behavior Surveillance: United States, 2005. *MMWR Morb Mortal Wkly Rep*. 2006;55:1–108
58. Centers for Disease Control and Prevention. Trends in HIV-related risk behaviors among high school students—United States, 1991–2005. *MMWR Morb Mortal Wkly Rep*. 2006;55:851–854
59. Buhi ER, Goodson P. Predictors of adolescent sexual behavior and intention: a theory-guided systematic review. *J Adolesc Health*. 2007;40:4–21
60. Nonnemaker JM, McNeely CA, Blumm RW; National Longitudinal Study of Adolescent Health. Public and private domains of religiosity and adolescent health risk behaviors: evidence from the National Longitudinal Study of Adolescent Health. *Soc Sci Med*. 2003;57:2049–2054
61. Crockett LJ, Bingham CR, Chopak JS, Vicary JR. Timing of first sexual intercourse: the role of social control, social learning, and problem behavior. *J Youth Adolesc*. 1996;25:89–111
62. Ott MA, Millstein SG, Ofner S, Halpern-Felsher BL. Greater expectations: adolescents' positive motivations for sex. *Perspect Sex Reprod Health*. 2006;38:84–89
63. Gebhardt WA, Kuyper L, Greunsven G. Need for intimacy in relationships and motives for sex as determinants of adolescent condom use. *J Adolesc Health*. 2003;33:154–164
64. Rosenthal SL, Von Ranson KM, Cotton S, Biro FM, Mills L, Succop PA. Sexual initiation: predictors and developmental trends. *Sex Transm Dis*. 2001;28:527–532
65. Parsons JT, Halkitis PN, Bimbi D, Borkowski T. Perceptions of the benefits and costs associated with condom use and unprotected sex among late adolescent college students. *J Adolesc*. 2000;23:377–391
66. Guttmacher Institute. U.S. teenage pregnancy statistics: national and state trends and trends by race and ethnicity. Available at: www.guttmacher.org/pubs/2006/09/12/USTPstats.pdf. Accessed October 8, 2007; 2006

67. Ventura SJ, Abma JC, Mosher WD, Henshaw S. Estimated pregnancy rates for the United States, 1990–2000: an update. *Natl Vital Stat Rep.* 2004;52(23):1–9
68. Hamilton BE, Martin JA, Ventura SJ. Births: preliminary data for 2005. *Natl Vital Stat Rep.* 2007;55(11):1–18
69. Hamilton BE, Ventura SJ. Fertility and abortion rates in the United States, 1960–2002. *Int J Androl.* 2006;29:34–45
70. Santelli J, Morrow B, Anderson JE, Lindberg LD. Contraceptive use and pregnancy risk among U.S. high school students: 1991–2003. *Perspect Sex Reprod Health.* 2006;38:106–111
71. Santelli JS, Lindberg LD, Finer LB, Singh S. Explaining recent declines in adolescent pregnancy in the United States: the contribution of abstinence and improved contraceptive use. *Am J Public Health.* 2007;97:150–156
72. Jaccard J, Dodge T, Dittus P. Do adolescents want to avoid pregnancy? Attitudes toward pregancy as predictors of pregnancy. *J Adolesc Health.* 2003;33:79–83
73. Bruckner H, Martin A, Bearman PS. Ambivalence and pregnancy: adolescents' attitudes, contraceptive use, and pregnancy. *Perspect Sex Reprod Health.* 2004;36:248–257
74. Boardman LA, Allsworth J, Phipps MG, Lapane KL. Risk factors for unintended versus intended rapid repeat pregnancies among adolescents. *J Adolesc Health.* 2006;39:597.e1–597.e8
75. Unger JB, Molina GB, Teran L. Perceived consequences of teenage childbearing among adolescent girls in an urban sample. *J Adolesc Health.* 2000;26:205–212
76. Olausson PO, Haglund B, Weitoft GR, Cnattingius S. Teenage childbearing and long-term socioeconomic consequences: a case study in Sweden. *Fam Plann Perspect.* 2001;33:70–74
77. Grogger J, Broners S. The socioeconomic consequences of teenage childbearing: findings from a natural experiment. *Fam Plann Perspect.* 1993;25:156–161, 174
78. Meade CS, Ickovics JR. Systematic review of sexual risk among pregnant and mothering teens in the USA: pregnancy as an opportunity for integrated prevention of STD and repeat pregnancy. *Soc Sci Med.* 2005;60:661–678
79. Birkeland R, Thompson JK, Phares V. Adolescent motherhood and postpartum depression. *J Clin Child Adolesc Psychol.* 2005;34:292–300
80. Gilbert W, Jandial D, Field N, Bigelow P, Danielsen B. Birth outcomes in teenage pregnancies. *J Matern Fetal Neonatal Med.* 2004;16:265–270
81. Menacker F, Martin JA, MacDorman MF, Ventura SJ. Births to 10–14 year-old mothers, 1990–2002: trends and health outcomes. *Natl Vital Stat Rep.* 2004;53(7):1–18
82. Kirby D. *Emerging Answers: Research Findings on Programs to Reduce Teen Pregnancy (Summary).* Washington, DC: National Campaign to Prevent Teen Pregnancy; 2001
83. Biro FM, Rosenthal SL. Psychological sequelae of sexually transmitted diseases in adolescents. *Obstet Gynecol Clin North Am.* 1992;19:209–218
84. Aral SO, Holmes KK. Epidemiology of sexual behavior and sexually transmitted diseases. In: Holmes KK, Mardh PM, Sparling PF, et al, eds. *Sexually Transmitted Diseases.* 2nd ed. New York, NY: McGraw-Hill; 1990:19–36
85. Centers for Disease Control and Prevention. Sexually transmitted treatment guidelines: 2006. *MMWR Morb Mortal Wkly Rep.* 2006;55:1–94
86. Weinstock H, Berman S, Cates W. Sexually transmitted diseases among American youth: incidence and prevalence estimates, 2000. *Perspect Sex Reprod Health.* 2004;36:6–10
87. Centers for Disease Control and Prevention. *Trends in Reportable Sexually Transmitted Diseases in the United States, 2005: National Surveillance Data for Chlamydia, Gonorrhea, and Syphilis.* Atlanta, GA: Centers for Disease Control Prevention; 2006
88. Dunne EF, Unger ER, Sternberg M, et al. Prevalence of HPV infection among females in the United States. *JAMA.* 2007;297:813–819
89. Auslander BA, Biro FM, Rosenthal SL. Genital herpes in adolescents. *Semin Pediatr Infect Dis.* 2005;16:24–30
90. Xu F, Sternberg MR, Kottiri BJ, et al. Trends in herpes simplex virus type 1 and type 2 seroprevalence in the United States. *JAMA.* 2006;296:964–973

91. Centers for Disease Control and Prevention. *HIV/AIDS Surveillance Report, 2005*. Atlanta, GA: US Department of Health and Human Services, Centers for Disease Control and Prevention; 2006
92. Boonstra H. Campaign to accelerate microbicide development for STD prevention gets under way. *Guttmacher Rep on Public Policy*. 2000;3:3–5
93. Aral SO. Sexually transmitted diseases: magnitude, determinants and consequences. *Int J STD AIDS*. 2001;12:211–215
94. Stagno S, Whitley RJ. Herpesvirus infections in neonates and children: cytomegalovirus and herpes simplex virus. In: Holmes KK, Sparling PF, Mardh PM, et al, eds. *Sexually Transmitted Diseases*. 3rd ed. New York, NY: McGraw-Hill; 1999:1191–1212
95. Nahmias AJ, Josey WE, Naib ZM, Freeman MG, Fernandez RJ, Wheeler JH. Perinatal risk associated with maternal genital herpes simplex virus infection. *Am J Obstet Gynecol*. 1971; 110:825–837
96. Hutto C, Arvin A, Jacobs R. Intrauterine herpes simplex virus infections. *J Pediatr*. 1987;110: 97–101
97. Corey L, Wald A, Celum C, Quinn TC. The effects of herpes simplex virus-2 on HIV-1 acquisition and transmission: a review of two overlapping epidemics. *J Acquire Immun Defic Syndr*. 2004;35:435–445
98. Shrier LA, Harris SK, Beardslee WR. Temporal associations between depressive symptoms and self-reported sexually transmitted disease among adolescents. *Arch Pediatr Adolesc Med*. 2002; 156:599–606
99. Baker JG, Succop PA, Boehner CW, Biro FM, Stanberry LR, Rosenthal SL. Adolescent girl's coping with an STD: not enough problem solving and too much self-blame. *J Pediatr Adolesc Gynecol*. 2001;14:85–88

Development of Intimate Relationships in Adolescence

Marissa Raymond, MPH[a], Marina Catallozzi, MD[a,b], Alison J. Lin, MPH[a], Owen Ryan, MPH, MIA[a], Vaughn I. Rickert, PsyD*[a,b]

[a]*Heilbrunn Department of Population and Family Health, Mailman School of Public Health, Columbia University, 60 Haven Avenue, New York, NY 10032, USA*

[b]*Department of Pediatrics, College of Physicians and Surgeons, Columbia University, 630 West 168th Street, New York, NY 10032, USA*

Although intimacy and romantic relationships occur between same-sex or -gender individuals with nonheterosexual sexual orientations, we focus largely on intimate and romantic relationships between young men and women in a heterocentric context because of the predominance of studies conducted with heterosexual youth and the lack of research on intimacy development in lesbian, gay, bisexual, and transgender youth. Similarly, in this article we use a binary definition of gender because of the profound lack of data about intimacy among transgender and non–gender-conforming youth. In addition, we noted significantly fewer studies about young men's experiences with intimacy than that of young women. Additional research is required on young men, lesbian, gay, bisexual, and transgender youth, as well as transgender and non–gender-conforming youth. In this article we report only on available data.

Intimacy in friendships, romances, and family relationships proceeds through a developmental continuum during adolescence. In late childhood (generally defined as ages 7–9 years), young people interact primarily with same-sex peers[2] and are greatly attached to their parents.[3] In early adolescence (defined here and in most research as ages 10–14 years), boys and girls report decreasing attachment to their parents[3] and establish opposite-gender friendships, socializing in mixed-gender crowds and group dating before progressing to dyadic interactions.[3–5]

---

*Corresponding author.
E-mail address: vir2002@columbia.edu (V. I. Rickert).

Copyright © 2007 American Academy of Pediatrics. All rights reserved. ISSN 1934-4287

Initial romantic relationships are intense and usually involve expressions of affection (most commonly sexual, inclusive of kissing, fondling, and sometimes sexual intercourse).[6] Collins defined romantic relationships as voluntary and ongoing interactions that are acknowledged by both members of a dyad. Several researchers have examined the developmental context of adolescent romantic relationships, specifically how previous attachment and relationships with family and peers impact romantic relationships. For example, Collins[6,7] reported an increase in dating from 25% in 12-year-olds to 75% in 17- and 18-year-olds. Similarly, adolescents 16 years of age and older reported longer relationships than their 14- to 15-year-old peers. Moreover, early adolescents tend to choose partners who will afford them greater social status and higher approval among peers, whereas older adolescents are more likely to look for partners with compatible attributes.[6,8,9]

Relationships with peers, family, and romantic partners build on one another as adolescents develop the skills to engage in young adult romantic relationships. Although this progression seems straightforward, many factors contribute to the relative success of adolescents' relationships and emotional health.

Figure 1 shows the developmental framework of the progression of intimacy. It also suggests the times of risk for particular forms of interpersonal violence that are further discussed by Lin et al.[10]

EARLY ADOLESCENCE

One of the main tasks of social development in early adolescence is the transition from dependence on and trust in parents to increased intimacy with peers.

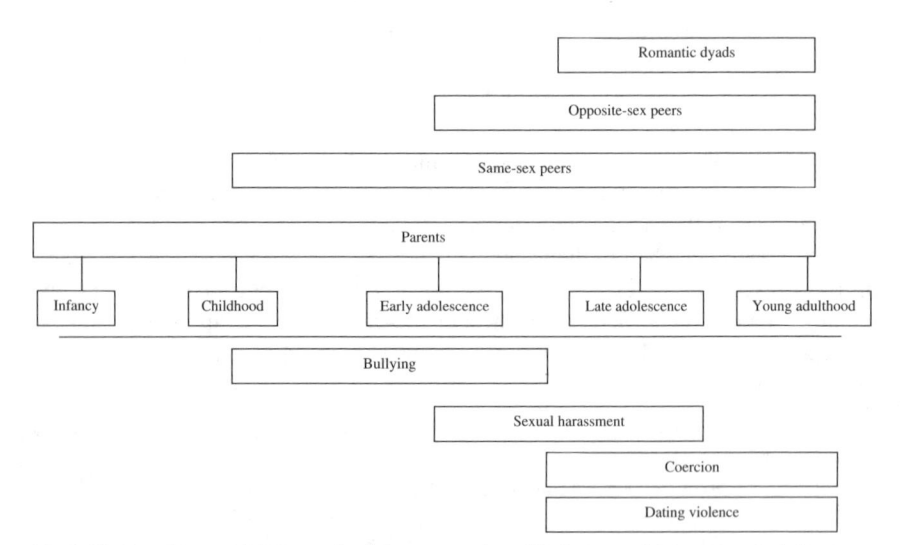

Fig 1 The developmental framework of the progression of intimacy and interpersonal violence.

Intimacy here is defined as a relationship with a person whom the adolescent relies on, talks to, confides in, and trusts. Girls report higher levels of attachment, support, trust, and communication with their friends than boys.[3,4,11–13] The friendships established in late childhood affect popularity among same- and opposite-gender peers into early adolescence.[14] Ultimately, these peer networks influence the course and direction of romantic relationships developed in late adolescence.

Family relationships are among the earliest relationships that children and early adolescents learn to navigate and change. For example, attachment to and communication with parents decline between fourth and sixth grade with a parallel decline in parental trust from fourth to eighth grade.[3] By the eighth grade, adolescents turn to peers to fulfill many of their attachment needs.[3] As an alternative to theories of increasing conflict with parents, several researchers have theorized an "atmosphere of continued connectedness" during adolescence to describe these changes.[15,16] These researchers purport that close or intimate relationships are interrelated over time and that parent-child relationships support and prepare youth for close friendships. The new and increased intimacy with peers further prepares youth for entering into romantic relationships. It is this secure foundation in family relationships and friendships that allows many adolescents to progress to other intimate relationships.[17,18]

Intimate friendships, like family relationships, contribute to healthy romantic relationship development; however, friendships can also have negative dimensions. Parker et al[19] found that friendship jealousy occurs most frequently among adolescent girls and those adolescents with low self-worth. Loneliness and adjustment difficulties are associated with higher levels of jealousy. Although high peer acceptance and higher-quality friendships in early adolescence are often perceived as positive, they are also associated with early initiation of romantic relationships and may mediate an increased number of sexual partners by late adolescence.[17,20] In some settings, peers may explicitly pressure adolescent girls into early sexual experimentation,[21] and it is believed that the same occurs with adolescent boys. Despite these negative aspects of early adolescent friendships, it is important to note that attachment to peers and parents is correlated with a higher degree of life satisfaction throughout early adolescence.[22]

The time that adolescents spend with or thinking about opposite-gender peers (both in friendships and romantic relationships) increases gradually over early adolescence, especially among adolescent girls.[13,23] As a consequence, early adolescent girls develop larger opposite-gender peer networks than boys.[13] These networks increase opposite-gender peer exposure and may contribute to the development of romantic relationships. Large opposite-gender peer networks are linked with greater amounts of self-disclosure, support, and longer romantic relationships among early adolescents.[13] Girls who maintain opposite-gender friendships also benefit from greater satisfaction with their bodies than girls without opposite-gender friends.[24]

As peer networks composed of a combination of young men and women increase, adolescents progress to dyadic dating.[21,24] Dating provides both companionship and support and is associated with a positive sense of self.[20] Early romantic relationships also provide opportunities to develop positive interpersonal skills and coping mechanisms for later relationships.[25]

Just as there are some negative aspects of adolescent friendships, there are also some negative effects of early adolescent romantic relationships, including poor academic performance among girls[23,26] and an increased risk of depression. Researchers have noted an increased risk for depression for adolescents, particularly girls, in romantic relationships. Similarly, youth who are not attracted to the opposite gender or who are questioning their sexual orientation are also at greater risk for depression and suicide.[27,28] Although less research exists specifically on boys, romantic relationships likely impact their social outcomes and mental health as well. Low self-esteem and antisocial behaviors also occur in certain groups of romantically involved adolescents, particularly those who are unpopular and those who have dated extensively at a young age.[28,29] Friendship neglect is another common byproduct of early adolescent romance. One study found that 53% of ninth-grade girls and 32% of ninth-grade boys reported previous neglect by a best friend who was preoccupied with a romantic relationship.[30] Neglect can place strain on the friendship and translate into jealously, anger, and pain for the neglected teen, with corresponding feelings of guilt for the romantically involved teen.[30] It takes time for adolescents to learn how to balance the needs of their peers and romantic partners. With increasing experience, adolescents gain coping skills that reduce their stress and increase the intimacy and duration of both their friendships and romantic relationships.[25]

LATE ADOLESCENCE

In late adolescence, the period between age 15 and the early 20s, young men and women further develop their relationships with opposite-gender peers and romantic partners.[12,25,31] As might be expected, friendships provide support for and have a positive impact on late adolescents. For example, young men and women who report a high degree of social support from peers in late adolescence also report a high degree of social acceptance, friendship competence, and romantic compeence.[32] In a study of urban, black, high-risk teens, stable attachment to peers was associated with fewer depressive symptoms and lower levels of stress, alcohol use, marijuana use, violent behavior, and delinquency. These subjects also reported greater success in school and rated school as more important than adolescents with less stable attachments.[33] However, stable, supportive peer and romantic relationships do not occur uniformly among adolescents. Miller et al[33] also found that <50% of participants reported having secure friendships. Another study of ethnically diverse participants found that adolescents only retain 34% to 50% of peers in their close-friendship groups each year throughout high school.[31]

Characteristics of friendships vary by gender. As with early adolescents, older-adolescent girls exhibit higher levels of positive friendship elements such as responsiveness, self-disclosure, and positive affect than young men.[12,31,34] Although young men and women rate their same-sex friendships as equal in quality, young men demonstrate higher levels of criticism and conflict at this age in their relationships than young women.[34] Adolescent boys may compensate for these relationship differences by drawing greater support from adults, particularly parents.[35] Although friendships between adolescent girls can be rich with support and positivity, these relationships may include negative consequences such as verbal assault, exclusive behaviors, and bullying and coercion.

Friendship demographics change in late adolescence. Teens continue same-sex friendships into late adolescence and report knowing their same-sex friends longer than their opposite-gender friends.[12] However, opposite-gender friendships become increasingly prevalent and important in late adolescence.[12,13,31] By the end of adolescence, opposite-gender friendships surpass same-sex friendship in cohesion and closeness.[12] It is not surprising, then, that late adolescents, especially young women, report spending or intending to spend more time with their opposite-gender peers than they did in their early adolescence.[13,23,36] Friendships and opposite-gender peer networks may be of particular importance for adolescent boys in same-sex romantic pairings. For example, it has been suggested that young gay men were less attached to romantic partners than their heterosexual peers but more attached to opposite-gender friends.[37] Thus, gay youth may seek and require a different peer-support structure than their heterosexual counterparts.

Opposite-gender friendships contribute to adolescent romantic relationship development. The peer network seems to be larger for adolescents who have romantic pairings; thus, teens who date seem to have more friends. Connolly and Johnson reported that youth in romantic dyads were more likely to have large peer networks, a greater number of friends of the opposite gender, and more friends outside of school. This expanded peer network is thought to support more successful romantic pairings.[38] In addition, the size of the opposite-gender peer network that an adolescent builds predicts his or her romantic relationship status[31,38] and correlates with some characteristics of his or her romantic relationships.[13] For example, 15-year-olds with large opposite-gender friendship networks have relationships that are characterized with more self-disclosure and support than adolescents with smaller opposite-gender peer networks.[13] By 18 years of age, adolescents with large opposite-gender friendship networks also report their romantic relationships as being longer in duration and having compatibility, friendship, and trust compared with adolescents with smaller opposite-gender networks[13]; however, these relationship qualities also might be influenced by the changes in peer networks that result from previous romantic connections.[31]

Romantic relationships later in adolescence are important, because they influence an adolescent's emotional health and shape his or her future relationships.[31] Adolescents can obtain many benefits from romantic relationships including gaining support from their romantic partners, gaining a more positive self-image, and obtaining the social skills necessary to negotiate future peer and romantic relationships.[25,39] With increased dating experience, older adolescents learn to discuss relationship challenges with their romantic partners and peers, which leads to a decline in relationship stresses.[25] These strategies for coping with romantic stress are linked to greater intimacy, affection, and duration of relationships in late adolescence despite a slight increase in romantic relationship conflict.[25]

Although dating benefits adolescents in many ways, it also poses some risks particular to older teens. Young women and adolescents in low-intimacy relationships are at higher risk for depression relative to young men and peers in high-intimacy relationships.[26,40] However, as adolescents transition into longer steady relationships, there is a corresponding decrease in depressive symptoms.[39] Similarly, dating multiple casual partners is a risk factor for experimentation with alcohol. Again, after the transition to steady relationships, associations between dating and alcohol use, as well as other minor delinquencies, decrease.[39] In the short term, dating can be associated with risk behaviors, but long-term stable relationships diminish these risks.

As adolescent relationships increase in quality and duration, they may increase in the level of sexual involvement.[39] In some cases, older adolescents engage in sexual activity in an effort to increase relationship intimacy and security, whereas other adolescents use sexual activity outside of committed relationships to increase their feelings of power and to gain status among their peers.[41-43] Some researchers report that young men seek sexual pleasure but struggle to develop emotional intimacy, whereas young women focus on developing both emotional and sexual intimacy.[43-45]

Perceptions of peers' sexual activities are strongly associated with an adolescent's sexual activity. For example, most adolescents who engage in oral sex are likely to report that their best friends had also engaged in oral sex; in contrast, adolescents who did not report engaging in oral sex are likely to report that their best friends also abstained from it.[42] Similarly, adolescents in networks of religious friends were less likely to engage in sexual intercourse than their peers with nonreligious networks.[46] The number of sexual partners a teen has by late adolescence is mediated directly by experimentation with alcohol and indirectly by early initiation of romantic relationships and popularity with peers.[20] The age difference between partners also influences initiation of intercourse. Adolescents with older partners are at particularly high risk for early sexual activity (typically defined as sexual intercourse before 14 years of age).[47]

Dating affects many aspects of adolescents' lives, including family relationships and friendships. In contrast to early adolescence, dating can actually improve friendships among older adolescents. That is, older teens who date casually report higher disclosure, greater feelings of closeness, and lower conflict with their best friends relative to nondaters or adolescents in steady relationships.[39,48] Young women in exclusive dating relationships may spend less time with their best friends, but they report that this change does not significantly affect the quality of their friendships.[48]

A great deal of emphasis has been placed recently on the impact of parents/families on adolescent sexual activity. One study conducted among minority adolescents who were sexual delayers (adolescents who intended to delay sex for at least 1 year) versus anticipators (adolescents who intended to have sex within the next year) demonstrated that the delayers rated their mothers as more responsive in discussing sex. In addition, the effect of sexually active peers on the adolescent's intention to have sex was buffered by a mother who was more responsive.[49] Similar findings have been reported among other high-risk populations with greater levels of family connectedness (eg, increased probability of never having had sex, lower rates of sex without a condom, less involvement in pregnancy, and, for young women, delayed initiation of sex and sexual risk-taking behaviors).[50] When using nationally representative samples, parental connectedness was found to be associated with low sexual risks in those adolescents who had supportive friends. In contrast, adolescents with supportive friends alone did not have lower sexual risk.[51]

Parents/families and peers also serve as sources of information about romantic relationships. Wood et al[52] examined sources of romantic relationship information, perceptions of information, and the influence of the source of information on the adolescent. Although they did not assess the specific types of information that adolescents received from different sources, data suggested that adolescents draw on a variety of sources to improve their understanding of romantic relationships. Specifically, girls received information about dating from several sources (rather than a large amount from 1 source). In contrast, boys obtained most of their information from the young women they dated. Although adolescents felt the most comfortable obtaining information from peers, they felt that the most reliable information came from adults such as sex educators (mostly teachers) or their parents. Regardless of these findings, reliability does not affect who has the most influence on their behavior or choices; peers still seem to have the most impact.

Roche et al[53] examined whether parental style affected sexual activity among a large, nationally representative sample. Their data suggest that the context of the family, specifically their neighborhood, has the strongest effect on sexual activity. Across all socioeconomic environments, families in which parents did not enforce rules regarding activity outside of the home were associated with youth engaged in higher levels of sexual activity. When parents did enforce rules on activities outside the home, the largest impact was noted in more socioeconomically disadvantaged neighborhoods.

CLINICAL IMPLICATIONS

Although we have discussed the typical development of healthy relationships, not all adolescents progress on the same, relatively safe trajectory. Clinicians promote healthy intimacy development by asking adolescent patients about their relationships with family, friends, and romantic interests. These questions can be a starting point for additional discussion and help to screen and identify adolescents who require additional support in their relationship choices.

The development of intimacy in friendships, romantic relationships, and family relationships occurs throughout adolescence. The skills that early adolescents gain with family members and friends translate into the strategies that they use to build relationships in late adolescence and early adulthood. Certain social factors can facilitate and alternatively impair the development of healthy romantic relationships (Table 1). Thus, those who create programmatic efforts that are designed to positively impact adolescent romantic relationships must consider the importance of healthy parental relationships with adolescents, as well as preparing parents to support their adolescents' romantic relationships. Moreover, the influence of peers cannot be overlooked, and effective peer education programs may assist in disseminating accurate and protective information for adolescents who are exploring relationships. Clinicians must be aware of the normal intimacy developmental continuum and screen for healthy and unhealthy family, peer, and romantic relationships in all adolescent patients. Adolescents want

Table 1
Influences on adolescent romantic relationships

Facilitatators
  Popularity among peers
  Supportive friendships
  Stable attachments
  Parent connectedness in infancy, childhood, and throughout adolescence
  Presence and size (larger) of mixed-gender peer network
  A limited number of supportive and healthy midadolescent romantic relationships
Impedances
  Jealousy among peers
  Peer pressure for early sexual initiation
  Lack of stable attachments, supportive friendships, or parent connectedness
  Early and excessive romantic relationships

healthy intimate romantic and peer relationships, and health care providers can assist them in developing the needed skills and support to help achieve those relationships.

REFERENCES

1. Sullivan HS. *The Interpersonal Theory of Psychiatry.* New York, NY: W. W. Norton & Company; 1953
2. Furman W. The emerging field of adolescent romantic relationships. *Curr Dir Psychol Sci.* 2002;11:177–180
3. Nickerson AB, Nagle RJ. Parent and peer attachment in late childhood and early adolescence. *J Early Adolesc.* 2005;25:223–249
4. Connolly J, Craig W, Goldberg A, Pepler D. Conceptions of cross-sex friendships and romantic relationships in early adolescence. *J Youth Adolesc.* 1999;28:481–494
5. Connolly J, Craig W, Goldberg A, Pepler D. Mixed-gender groups, dating, and romantic relationships in early adolescence. *J Res Adolesc.* 2004;14:185–207
6. Collins WA. More than myth: the developmental significance of romantic relationships during adolescence. *J Res Adolesc.* 2003;13:1–24
7. Carver K, Joyner K, Udry JRE. National estimates of adolescent romantic relationships. In: Florsheim P, ed. *Adolescent Romantic Relations and Sexual Behavior: Theory, Research, and Practical Implications.* Mahwah, NJ: Erlbaum; 2003:23–56
8. Roscoe B, Diana MS, Brooks RH. Early, middle, and late adolescents views on dating and factors influencing partner selection. *Adolescence.* 1987;22:59–68
9. Zani B. Dating and interpersonal relationships in adolescence. In: Jackson S, Rodriguez-Tome H, eds. *Adolescence and Its Social Worlds.* Hillsdale, NJ: Erlbaum; 1993:95–120
10. Lin AJ, Raymond M, Catallozzi M, Ryan O, Rickert VI. Relationship violence in adolescence. *Adolesc Med.* 2007;18:530–543
11. Bradley LA, Flannagan D, Fuhrman R. Judgment biases and characteristics of friendships of Mexican American and Anglo-American girls and boys. *J Early Adolesc.* 2001;21:405–424
12. Johnson HD. Gender, grade, and relationship differences in emotional closeness within adolescent friendships. *Adolescence.* 2004;39:243–255
13. Feiring C. Other-sex friendship networks and the development of romantic relationships in adolescence. *J Youth Adolesc.* 1999;28:495–512
14. Zettergren P. Childhood peer status as predictor of midadolescence peer situation and social adjustment. *Psychol Sch.* 2005;42:745–757
15. Rice KG, Mulkeen P. Relationships with parents and peers: a longitudinal-study of adolescent intimacy. *J Adolesc Res.* 1995;10:338–357
16. Montemayor R, Flannery D. Parent-adolescent relations in middle and late adolescence. In: Petersen A, Brooks-Gunn J, eds. *Encyclopedia of Adolescence.* New York, NY: Garland; 1991:729–734
17. Collins WA, Laursen B. Changing relationships, changing youth: interpersonal contexts of adolescent development. *J Early Adolesc.* 2004;24:55–62
18. Parke RD, Buriel R. Socialization in the family: ethnic and ecological perspectives. In: Damon W, Eisenberg N, eds. *Handbook of Child Psychology: Social, Emotional, and Personality Development.* Vol 3. New York, NY: John Wiley; 1998:463–552
19. Parker JG, Low CM, Walker AR, Gamm BK. Friendship jealousy in young adolescents: individual differences and links to sex, self-esteem, aggression, and social adjustment. *Dev Psychol.* 2005;41:235–250
20. Zimmer-Gembeck MJ, Siebenbruner J, Collins WA. A prospective study of intraindividual and peer influences on adolescents' heterosexual romantic and sexual behavior. *Arch Sex Behav.* 2004;33:381–394
21. O'Sullivan LF, Meyer-Bahlburg HFL. African-American and Latina inner-city girls' reports of romantic and sexual development. *J Soc Pers Relat.* 2003;20:221–238

22. Nickerson AB, Nagle RJ. The influence of parent and peer attachments on life satisfaction in middle childhood and early adolescence. *Soc Indicators Res.* 2004;66:35–60
23. Richards MH, Crowe PA, Larson R, Swarr A. Developmental patterns and gender differences in the experience of peer companionship during adolescence. *Child Dev.* 1998;69:154–163
24. Compian L, Gowen LK, Hayward C. Peripubertal girls' romantic and platonic involvement with boys: associations with body image and depression symptoms. *J Res Adolesc.* 2004;14:23–47
25. Nieder T, Seiffge-Krenke I. Coping with stress in different phases of romantic development. *J Adolesc.* 2001;24:297–311
26. Joyner K, Udry JR. You don't bring me anything but down: adolescent romance and depression. *J Health Soc Behav.* 2000;41:369–391
27. Garofalo R, Katz E. Health care issues of gay and lesbian youth. *Curr Opin Pediatr.* 2001;13:298–302
28. Brendgen M, Vitaro F, Doyle AB, Markiewicz D, Bukowski WM. Same-sex peer relations and romantic relationships during early adolescence: interactive links to emotional, behavioral, and academic adjustment. *Merrill Palmer Q J Dev Psychol.* 2002;48:77–103
29. Zimmer-Gembeck MJ, Siebenbruner J, Collins WA. Diverse aspects of dating: associations with psychosocial functioning from early to middle adolescence. *J Adolesc.* 2001;24:313–336
30. Roth MA, Parker JG. Affective and behavioral responses to friends who neglect their friends for dating partners: influences of gender, jealousy and perspective. *J Adolesc.* 2001;24:281–296
31. Connolly J, Furman W, Konarski R. The role of peers in the emergence of heterosexual romantic relationships in adolescence. *Child Dev.* 2000;71:1395–1408
32. Laursen B, Furman W, Mooney KS. Predicting interpersonal competence and self-worth from adolescent relationships and relationship networks: variable-centered and person-centered perspectives. *Merrill Palmer Q J Dev Psychol.* 2006;52:572–600
33. Miller AL, Notaro PC, Zimmerman MA. Stability and change in internal working models of friendship: associations with multiple domains of urban adolescent functioning. *J Soc Pers Relat.* 2002;19:233–259
34. Brendgen M, Markiewicz D, Doyle AB, Bukowski WM. The relations between friendship quality, ranked-friendship preference, and adolescents' behavior with their friends. *Merrill Palmer Q J Dev Psychol.* 2001;47:395–415
35. Colarossi LG. Adolescent gender differences in social support: structure, function, and provider type. *Soc Work Res.* 2001;25:233–241
36. Strough J, Covatto AM. Context and age differences in same- and other-gender peer preferences. *Soc Dev.* 2002;11:346–361
37. Diamond LM, Dube EM. Friendship and attachment among heterosexual and sexual-minority youths: does the gender of your friend matter? *J Youth Adolesc.* 2002;31:155–166
38. Connolly JA, Johnson AM. Adolescents' romantic relationships and the structure and quality of their close interpersonal ties. *Pers Relat.* 1996;3:185–195
39. Davies PT, Windle M. Middle adolescents' dating pathways and psychosocial adjustment. *Merrill Palmer Q J Dev Psychol.* 2000;46:90–118
40. Williams S, Connolly J, Segal ZV. Intimacy in relationships and cognitive vulnerability to depression in adolescent girls. *Cognit Ther Res.* 2001;25:477–496
41. Schachner DA, Shaver PR. Attachment dimensions and sexual motives. *Pers Relat.* 2004;11:179–195
42. Prinstein MJ, Meade CS, Cohen GL. Adolescent oral sex, peer popularity, and perceptions of best friends' sexual behavior. *J Pediatr Psychol.* 2003;28:243–249
43. Ott MA, Millstein SG, Ofner S, Halpern-Felsher BL. Greater expectations: adolescents' positive motivations for sex. *Perspect Sex Reprod Health.* 2006;38:84–89
44. Harper GW, Gannon C, Watson SE, Catania JA, Dolcini MM. The role of close friends in African American adolescents' dating and sexual behavior. *J Sex Res.* 2004;41:351–362
45. Korobov N, Thorne A. Intimacy and distancing: young men's conversations about romantic relationships. *J Adolesc Res.* 2006;21:27–55
46. Adamczyk A, Felson J. Friends' religiosity and first sex. *Soc Sci Res.* 2006;35:924–947

47. Marin BV, Kirby DB, Hudes ES, Coyle KK, Gomez CA. Boyfriends, girlfriends and teenagers' risk of sexual involvement. *Perspect Sex Reprod Health*. 2006;38:76–83
48. Kuttler AF, La Greca AM. Linkages among adolescent girls' romantic relationships, best friendships, and peer networks. *J Adolesc*. 2004;27:395–414
49. Fasula AM, Miller KS. African-American and Hispanic adolescents' intentions to delay first intercourse: parental communication as a buffer for sexually active peers. *J Adolesc Health*. 2006;38:193–200
50. Markham CM, Tortolero SR, Escobar-Chaves SL, Parcel GS, Harrist R, Addy RC. Family connectedness and sexual risk-taking among urban youth attending alternative high schools. *Perspect Sex Reprod Health*. 2003;35:174–179
51. Henrich CC, Brookmeyer KA, Shrier LA, Shahar G. Supportive relationships and sexual risk behavior in adolescence: an ecological-transactional approach. *J Pediat Psychol*. 2006;31:286–297
52. Wood E, Senn CY, Desmarais S, Park L, Verberg N. Sources of information about dating and their perceived influence on adolescents. *J Adolesc Res*. 2002;17:401–417
53. Roche KM, Mekos D, Alexander CS, Astone NM, Bandeen-Roche K, Ensminger ME. Parenting influences on early sex initiation among adolescents: how neighborhood matters. *J Fam Issues*. 2005;26:32–54

Parental Influences on Adolescent Sexual Behaviors

Richard Rupp, MD*, Susan L. Rosenthal, PhD

Department of Pediatrics, University of Texas Medical Branch, 301 University Boulevard, Galveston, TX 77555-1119, USA

As children mature, there are increasing numbers of influences on their development and behavioral choices. Often parents of teens feel worried that their influence is waning and being replaced by other influences, in particular peers and the media; however, this is in fact not entirely the case. Although peers do have an increasing effect on adolescents' lives, their influence is additive to the influence of parents. Adolescents are not different from adults in that they tend to seek the wisdom of those who are perceived as the experts. Adolescents typically see their parents as "experts" on issues of morals and values and on health-related matters; and their peers as "experts" on matters of personal taste such as hair and clothing styles.[1,2] In addition, research has demonstrated that relationships with parents can have an impact on the effectiveness of peer influence. For example, studies show that adolescents who communicated with their parents about sexual matters were less likely to be influenced by when their peers began having intercourse.[3,4] However, parenting style is related to the likelihood that parents will have a positive impact on their adolescents' sexual choices. Parents who use authoritative parenting are more likely to have psychosocially competent adolescents. Authoritative parenting is characterized by limit-setting which is responsive to the adolescent and his/her developmental level in the context of a warm and supportive relationship with good communication. In the following chapter, we will review the literature on adolescent sexual behavior as related to the following aspects of authoritative parenting; monitoring, communication, and modeling. Programs incorporating parents in an attempt to reduce adolescent sexual risk behaviors will be examined as well. Finally, we will relate the knowledge about parental attitudes and adolescent sexual development to a topic recently facing health care providers, the recommendation that adolescent girls all receive the HPV vaccine.

---

*Corresponding author.

E-mail address: rrupp@utmb.edu (R. Rupp).

Copyright © 2007 American Academy of Pediatrics. All rights reserved. ISSN 1934-4287

PARENTAL MONITORING

Parental monitoring involves parental knowledge of the child's whereabouts, activities, and associates, although the specifics of how monitoring is measured or described varies across studies. In most families, mothers know more than fathers about their adolescents' activities, and most fathers receive their information from the mother.[5,6] There is a developmental aspect of monitoring. As adolescents age, parents move from direct supervision by way of the physical presence of an adult to monitoring through knowledge of whom they are with and where they are. Although parental monitoring wanes with age, its positive effects persist well into late adolescence.[7-9]

Because monitoring usually occurs through active supervision or disclosure by the adolescent, it requires good communication between parent and child. The effectiveness, therefore, depends on the willingness of the teenager to freely disclose information.[10,11] The relationship between monitoring and parent-adolescent communication is complex. In itself, the act of monitoring communicates parental values and expectations. Adolescents reporting successful parental monitoring expressed cognitions significantly less favorable of initiating intercourse.[12] Thus, communication is an important aspect of monitoring and supervision and is discussed in "Parent-Adolescent Communication" below.

Some studies have indicated increased monitoring of girls compared with boys, but others have found no differences.[7,8,10,13,14] Likewise, the data on the effect of monitoring by gender have been mixed. One study showed that monitoring equally affects risk taking in both genders, whereas another study showed lower sexual risk-taking behaviors in well-monitored boys but no effect in girls.[11,15]

Monitoring, in and of itself, is likely insufficient to protect adolescents from unsafe situations and risky activities if parental rules are too permissive and the parents do not provide enough supervision. For example, 1 study found that permissive parental rules regarding curfew significantly differed between girls who were sexually experienced and those who were not. Those with looser curfews were more likely to have had sexual intercourse.[16] The number of areas in which parents had rules and the degree to which an adolescent was allowed to decide rules were significant predictors of the frequency of sexual intercourse. Greater freedom was associated with a higher frequency of intercourse.[17]

Parental monitoring has been demonstrated to lower the likelihood that an adolescent will engage in a variety of health-risk behaviors. With regards to sexual health, adolescents who describe their family as providing supervision were older at sexual initiation.[8,9,18,19] Not only are adolescents older when they initiate sex, but they are more likely to have the perception of the age at first intercourse as "just right" as opposed to "too early."[20] Among the sexually experienced, monitoring has been associated with having fewer risky partners, contraception use, and less frequent intercourse.[7,11,21,22] This relationship between monitoring and safer-sex practices is confirmed by fewer adverse outcomes. Less monitoring has been associated with a greater likelihood of testing positive for sexually transmitted infections and increased pregnancy rates.[5,23–26]

As noted in the introduction, parenting needs to be responsive to the developmental needs of adolescents. Parents need to prepare their children to become independent and capable of making healthy choices when they are not supervised. Indeed, expectations adjust as the adolescent ages, allowing for more freedom and the development of decision-making skills.[7,8] Adolescents often request an expansion of their boundaries by negotiating, in advance, to bend rules that surround curfews and adult supervision. Little is known about how this process occurs and its implication for the health and well-being of adolescents. In the 1 study that examined "negotiated unsupervised time," mixed results were found. On one hand, negotiated unsupervised time was found to be strongly associated with increased sexual activity but, on the other hand, it also was found to be related to sex-related protective behaviors (eg, condom use).[15] Clearly, a better understanding of this process is needed so that health care providers can support adolescents in their efforts to gain increasing independence without leading to health risk behaviors.

PARENT-ADOLESCENT COMMUNICATION

There is general agreement among professionals, parents, and adolescents that talking about sexuality within the family is important, and research supports the idea that more frequent and positive parent-adolescent communication is associated with better sexual outcomes such as later sexual initiation, encountering fewer partners, and better use of contraception.[21,27–30] The quality of the parent-adolescent relationship is paramount. Adolescent perceptions of problem communication and/or looser family ties were associated with increased sexual risk behaviors.[28] Adolescents who feel their parent to be supportive and open are more likely to incorporate the parent's message. For example, adolescents whose mother disclosed her experiences with sexuality and dating felt a sense of openness and connectedness and expressed more conservative adolescent attitudes regarding premarital sexual behavior.[31] Many studies have indicated that adolescents with better parental relationships, feelings of connectedness to the mother, or feeling that parents care have fewer risk behaviors.[21,32–37] Parents who were perceived as less supportive but still discussed sexual issues had adolescents who reported more sexual risk taking.[27] Thus, when a parent and adolescent are engaged in a hostile and unsupportive relationship, communication on sexual issues may have little impact because the interaction is likely to be poor.

The difficulty in studying communication lies in the fact that it is not a single construct. There are many aspects of communication that likely impact its effectiveness such as the timing, mode, and content. For example, talking to an adolescent about postponing the initiation of intercourse is ineffective when the adolescent is already sexually experienced (poor timing). The importance in timing was shown in a study in which discussing condom use before sexual debut was strongly associated with more frequent use at first intercourse and more frequent lifetime regular condom use.[38] The timing of communication and its relationship to causality is complex and may get obscured in cross-sectional data collection. Did the adolescent behavior induce certain communications from parents, or did parental communication produce particular behaviors in the adolescent? One group found that greater teen-parent communication was associated with increased odds of sex with an older partner relative to not having sex. They postulated that the greater communication occurred in response to riskier teen behaviors such as attending unsupervised parties, dating at a young age, or using drugs or alcohol.[39]

Accounting for the different modes of communication has challenged researchers as well. A study of pregnant Latina adolescents found that those whose mothers used more explicit terms when communicating about contraception and sexuality reported more confidence about using condoms and increased comfort in talking to partners about condoms.[40] Many studies have explored direct parent-adolescent communications through questions such as "have you and your mother discussed sex?" However, many messages are communicated indirectly through parents' off-the-cuff comments or reactions to events in everyday life. For example, an adolescent may gain insight into her mother's values by observing her expressing to others her disapproval of a family friend's out-of-wedlock pregnancy. Such indirect communication is often studied by looking at the adolescents' perceptions of their parents' values. Adolescent perception of maternal disapproval of involvement in sexual risk behaviors is associated with later initiation, having fewer partners, less frequent sexual activity, more negative attitudes toward teen pregnancy, and decreased teen pregnancy.[22,27,34,36,41] Of concern is that adolescent perceptions may be mistaken and "safer-sex" messages may be interpreted as approval of sexual activity. In 1 study, virgins who perceived maternal approval of birth control had an increased likelihood of sexual intercourse over the next 12 months but, at the same time, were also more likely to have used birth control.[35] Indeed, children may underestimate their parents' opposition to their engaging in sexual activities;[34,42] Parents should not take their child's understanding for granted; parents should spell out their values and expectations clearly.

The actual content of the conversation is important as well. Although parents and adolescents both feel that discussions on sexual issues are important, both groups tend to feel uneasy about discussing such matters. Mothers were more likely to communicate with their adolescent if they felt knowledgeable.[43] Few, if any, families cover all topics or issues surrounding sexuality. Common themes include the consequences of AIDS/sexually transmitted diseases or pregnancy and how to protect against them. Less frequently discussed are topics such as masturbation, wet dreams, sexual development, and choosing a sexual partner.[30,44] In addition, adolescent and parent perceptions of communication on sexual topics correlate only modestly. Parents often believed they were more communicative about sexual issues than their adolescent perceived them to be.[44] When such discussions do occur, they lead to a greater belief that parents are the best source about sex and decrease the likelihood of the adolescent being sexually experienced.[28]

It seems that more information is communicated from parents to daughters.[30,44] Mothers are the primary communicators about sexual matters for both sons and daughters. Parents are more likely to speak about sexual issues with their same-gender adolescent (ie, a mother is more likely to speak with her daughters than her sons). Topics such as contraception, condom use, physical development, and sexual pressure are likely to be discussed by same-gender pairs.[30,44]

MODELED BEHAVIORS IN THE FAMILY

Families communicate expectations regarding appropriate behavior not only through direct verbal communications with adolescents but also by their behavior. Both past and present behavior within the family seems to communicate values or, at least, is related to the actual behavior of adolescents. The elevated risk of pregnancy among adolescent girls whose mother had her first child as a teenager is well established.[29,45] Research has shown that both male and female adolescents with mothers who had their first pregnancy as a teenager are likely to have an earlier age of sexual initiation, even after controlling for family structure and socioeconomic status.[14,30,44] In a similar way, adolescents living with pregnant or parenting sisters are more likely to be sexually experienced and to have more permissive sexual attitudes.[29,46,47] It would be overly simplistic to state that repeat teen pregnancy within families is attributable solely to modeling. Socioeconomic status, family structure, social environment, and perhaps even genetics play significant roles. Household dynamics surrounding teen pregnancies are complicated. After delivery, families often face greater financial stress, along with the additional burden of infant care. Mothers of childbearing teens may give preferential treatment to their nonchildbearing children. On the other hand, the childbearing teen may gain stature and power within the household.[48,49] These stresses and changes in family dynamics impact the nonchildbearing siblings. Although the past behavior of mothers and siblings is not something that the health care provider (or the mother) can change, it can be used as a way to identify adolescents who may be at high risk and have special needs.

Although the issues are complex and difficult to sort out, it is to be expected that modeling does influence adolescent risk behaviors, because parents' behavior plays a fundamental role in defining what is normal for their children. Risky parental behavior (ie, smoking, drinking, and not using a seatbelt) is associated with risky adolescent behaviors that include smoking, drinking, delinquency, and a younger age at first coitus.[50] One study found that parental divorce with subsequent repartnering greatly increased the occurrence of sexual initiation of at-risk adolescent boys.[51] Another study of divorced mothers showed that the mother's dating behaviors (ie, increased frequency of dating, more date partners, and briefer period between divorce and dating) were associated with more permissive attitudes about sexuality among daughters and earlier sexual behaviors in both sons and daughters.[52] Parents should be educated and reminded that behaviors observed in the home around/within intimate relationships may be especially influential during adolescence when children are developing their own sexual identity.

PARENTING INTERVENTIONS

In recognition of the importance of family processes, several adolescent sexual health promotion programs incorporate parenting components. The parenting goals vary from program to program but include expanding parents' knowledge and awareness of sexual issues, increasing comfort levels, discussing sexual issues, improving communication skills, and encouraging monitoring and supervision. For large-scale interventions, one of the biggest obstacles is the competition with other events/issues in parents' busy lives in getting them to commit to participation. Attempts to involve parents have included not only the traditional parents-teens and parents-only sessions but also homework assignments that required parent participation to be completed by the adolescent, video productions for home family viewing, and newsletters mailed to parents.[27,53-55]

Although few of the programs have been rigorously evaluated, the overall results have been somewhat positive. Encouraging findings include increases in parent and child knowledge, parental satisfaction with the intervention, enhanced parent-adolescent communication, and short-term reductions in sexual risk behaviors.[54-58] In one of the best-evaluated studies, adolescents received either a skills-based HIV risk-reduction intervention alone or the same intervention coupled with a parent-child session delivered in the home that was designed to improve communication and monitoring. Those adolescents in the enhanced program reported greater self-efficacy for refusing high-risk behaviors and less intention to initiate sex. Six months after the program, the same youth reported significantly lower rates of sexual intercourse, sex without a condom, and alcohol and drug use.[59] However, these results were not sustained long-term. By 24 months there were no differences in sexual behaviors between the groups, except those who had the enhanced version were more likely to ask their partner if condoms were always used.[60] Because parenting evolves as adolescents mature, future research should study the extension of interventions through adolescence to strengthen parenting skills and boost parent-adolescent communication.

FAMILIES AND THE HPV VACCINE

The licensure of the first HPV vaccine brought to the forefront issues related to sexual mores and parenting. The vaccine is currently licensed by the Food and Drug Administration for the prevention of cervical cancer, dysplasia, and genital warts. Although it is licensed for girls down to the age of 9 years, the Centers for Disease Control and Prevention Advisory Committee on Immunization Practices targets the vaccine for girls 11 to 12 years old and recommends a "catch-up" vaccination for older girls who have not been vaccinated. These recommendations are supported by several leading medical organizations (eg, American Academy of Pediatrics, Society for Adolescent Medicine, American Academy of Family Physicians, American College of Obstetricians and Gynecologists).

Studies have shown that most parents desire to vaccinate their child and that it is the severity of the disease and effectiveness of the vaccine that matter, not the mode of disease transmission.[61,62] Mothers are interested in preventing cancer in their daughters. One study found that the addition of protection against genital warts was seen as somewhat trivial by some but did not make women less likely to want to vaccinate their daughters.[63]

Some mothers may have reservations about vaccinating at a young age. Some may feel that discussing the vaccine is too difficult with young girls who have little knowledge of sex. Others have expressed that this may be an ideal age, because the conversation can be avoided until their daughter is older.[63] Parents should be taught that communications about sexual issues should be recurring and should be altered to match the developmental maturity of the adolescent.

Concerned parents often wish to discuss the vaccine and its influence on adolescent sexual behavior with the health care provider. Parents may be hesitant to vaccinate, because they fear it may falsely lend tacit support to activities contrary to their moral values. Others have expressed concerns that the vaccine may increase the risk of acquiring other sexually transmitted infections (eg, HIV) by giving adolescents a false sense of security, leading to increased risk taking.[63] Studies of young adults have indicated that vaccination would not change their sexual behaviors.[64] Also, some professionals use the analogy of encouraging automobile seatbelt use, which is not known to encourage reckless driving.[65] Parents should be reminded what their life experience has already taught them: very few teenagers are dissuaded from sexual activity by fear of either sexually transmitted diseases or pregnancy. Parents who voice these concerns should be counseled to clearly communicate their values and expectations and to monitor and supervise their daughters.

CONCLUSION

This review of the literature reinforces the idea that parents influence the sexual health of their children. Parents should remain engaged and actively involved in their adolescents' lives to influence sexual risk-taking behavior. Parental monitoring and supervision are important avenues for keeping adolescents away from risky situations and activities while the teenager develops responsible decision-making skills. As adulthood approaches, monitoring relies increasingly on information shared by the adolescent. Parents should tailor discussions to the developmental level of the adolescent and should clearly define parental values and expectations. Maintaining an open, supportive relationship with the adolescent is important for enhancing communication and supervision. Parents should be cognizant that their own behaviors will influence their adolescents' beliefs and behaviors as well.

Thus, an important responsibility of health care providers is to offer parents guidance on developmentally appropriate methods of monitoring and communication about sexuality as a way to support adolescents' growth into healthy, sexually responsible adults.

REFERENCES

1. Steinberg L. *Adolescence*. 7th ed. New York, NY: McGraw Hill; 2005
2. Smetana JG, Asquith P. Adolescents' and parents' conceptions of parental authority and personal autonomy. *Child Dev*. 1994;65:1147–1162
3. Fasula AM, Miller KS. African-American and Hispanic adolescents' intentions to delay first intercourse: parental communication as a buffer for sexually active peers. *J Adolesc Health*. 2006;38:193–200
4. Whitaker DJ, Miller KS. Parent-adolescent discussions about sex and condoms: impact on peer influences of sexual risk behavior. *J Adolesc Res*. 2000;15:251–273
5. DiClemente RJ, Wingood GM, Crosby RA, et al. Parental monitoring: association with adolescents' risk behaviors. *Pediatrics*. 2001;107:1363–1368
6. Waizenhofer RN, Buchanan CM, Jackson-Newsom J. Mothers' and fathers' knowledge of adolescents' daily activities: its sources and its links with adolescent adjustment. *J Fam Psychol*. 2004;18:348–360
7. Rai AA, Stanton B, Wu Y, et al. Relative influences of perceived parental monitoring and perceived peer involvement on adolescent risk behaviors: an analysis of six cross-sectional data sets. *J Adolesc Health*. 2003;33:108–118
8. Li X, Feigelman S, Stanton B. Perceived parental monitoring and health risk behaviors among urban low-income African-American children and adolescents. *J Adolesc Health*. 2000;27:43–48
9. Li X, Stanton B, Feigelman S. Impact of perceived parental monitoring on adolescent risk behavior over 4 years. *J Adolesc Health*. 2000;27:49–56
10. Stattin H, Kerr M. Parental monitoring: a reinterpretation. *Child Dev*. 2000;71:1072–1085
11. Huebner AJ, Howell LW. Examining the relationship between adolescent sexual risk taking and perceptions of monitoring, communication and parenting styles. *J Adolesc Health*. 2003;33:71–78
12. Sieverding JA, Alder N, Witt S, Ellen J. The influence of parental monitoring on adolescent sexual initiation. *Arch Pediatr Adolesc Med*. 159:724–729
13. Jacobson KC, Crockett LJ. Parental monitoring and adolsecent adjustment: an ecological perspective. *J Res Adolesc*. 2000;10:65–97
14. Bonell C, Allen E, Strange V, et al. Influence of family type and parenting behaviours on teenage sexual behaviour and conceptions. *J Epidemiol Community Health*. 2006;60:502–506
15. Borawski EA, Ievers-Landis CE, Lovegreen LD, Trapl ES. Parental monitoring, negotiated unsupervised time and parental trust: the role of perceived parenting practices in adolescent health risk behaviors. *J Adolesc Health*. 2003;33:60–70

16. Ensminger ME. Sexual activity and problem behaviors among black, urban adolescents. *Child Dev.* 1990;61:2032–2046
17. Turner SL, Scott-Jones D. The influence of parental supervision and rules on black adolescent females' sexual activity. Presented at: fourth biennial meeting of the Society for Research On Adolescence; March 1992; Washington, DC
18. Rosenthal SL, Von Ranson KM, Cotton S, Biro FM, Mills L, Succop PA. Sexual initiation: predictors and developmental trends. *Sex Transm Dis.* 2001;28:527–532
19. Romer D, Stanton B, Galbraith J, Feigelman S, Black MM, Li X. Parental influence on adolescent sexual behavior in high-poverty settings. *Arch Pediatr Adolesc Med.* 1999;153:1055–1062
20. Cotton S, Mills L, Succop PA, Biro FM, Rosenthal SL. Adolescent girls' perceptions of the timing of their sexual initiation: "too young" or "just right." *J Adolesc Health.* 2004;34:453–458
21. Rose A, Koo HP, Bhasker B, Anderson K, White G, Jenkins R. The influence of primary caregivers on the sexual behavior of early adolescents. *J Adolesc Health.* 2005;37:135–144
22. McNeely C, Shew ML, Beuhring T, Sieving R, Miller B, Blum RW. Mothers' influence on the timing of first sex among 14- and 15- year-olds. *J Adolesc Health.* 2002;31:256–265
23. Bettinger JA, Celentano DD, Curriero FC, Adler NE, Millstein SG, Ellen JM. Does parental involvement predict new sexually transmitted diseases in female adolescents? *Arch Pediatr Adolesc Med.* 2004;158:666–670
24. Biglan A, Metzler CW, Wirt R, et al. Social and behavioral factors associated with high-risk sexual behavior among adolescents. *J Behav Med.* 1990;13:245–261
25. Crosby RA, DiClemente RJ, Wingood GM, et al. Low parental monitoring predicts subsequent pregnancy among African-American adolescent females. *J Pediatr Adolesc Gynecol.* 2002;15:43–46
26. Crosby RA, DiClemente RJ, Wingood GM, Lang DL, Harrington K. Infrequent parental monitoring predicts sexually transmitted infections among low income African-American adolescent females. *Arch Pediatr Adolesc Med.* 2003;157:169–173
27. Meschke LL, Bartholomae S, Zentall SR. Adolescent sexuality and parent-adolescent processes: promoting healthy teen choices. *J Adolesc Health.* 2002;31:264–279
28. Whitaker DJ, Miller KS, Clark LF. Reconceptualizing adolescent sexual behavior: beyond did they or didn't they? *Fam Plann Perspect.* 2000;32:111–117
29. Miller BC, Benson B, Galbraith KA. Family relationships and adolescent pregnancy risk: a research synthesis. *Dev Rev.* 2001;21:1–38
30. DiIorio C, Kelley M, Hockenberry-Eaton M. Communication about sexual issues: mothers, fathers and friends. *J Adolesc Health.* 1999;24:181–189
31. Romo LF, Lefkowitz ES, Sigman M, Au TK. A longitudinal study of maternal messages about dating and sexuality and their influence on Latino adolescents. *J Adolesc Health.* 2002;31:59–69
32. Aronowitz T, Morrison-Beedy D. Resilience to risk-taking behaviors in impoverished African American girls: the role of mother-daughter connectedness. *Res Nurs Health.* 2004;27:29–39
33. Parera N, Suris JC. Having a good relationship with their mother: a protective factor against sexual risk behavior among adolescent females? *Pediatr Adolesc Gynecol.* 2004;17:267–271
34. Dittus PJ, Jaccard J. Adolescents' perceptions of maternal disapproval of sex: relationship to sexual outcomes. *J Adolesc Health.* 2000;26:268–278
35. Jaccard J, Dittus PJ. Adolescent perceptions of maternal approval of birth control and sexual risk behavior. *Am J Public Health.* 2000;90:1426–1430
36. Jaccard J, Dodge T, Dittus P. Maternal discussions about pregnancy and adolescents, attitudes toward pregnancy. *J Adolesc Health.* 2003;33:84–87
37. Lammers C, Ireland M, Resnick M, Blum R. Influences on adolescents' decision to postpone onset of sexual intercourse: a survival analysis of virginity among youths aged 13 to 18 years. *J Adolesc Health.* 2000;26:42–48
38. Miller KS, Levin ML, Whitaker DJ, Xu X. Patterns of condom use among adolescents: the impact of mother-adolescent communication. *Am J Public Health.* 1998;88:1542–1544
39. Manlove JS, Ryan S, Franzetta K. Risk and protective factors associated with the transition to a first sexual relationship with an older partner. *J Adolesc Health.* 2007;40:135–143

40. Nadeem E, Romo LF, Sigman M. Knowledge about condoms among low-income pregnant Latina adolescents in relation to explicit maternal discussion of contraceptives. *J Adolesc Health*. 2006;39:119.e9–119.e15
41. Resnick MD, Bearman PS, Blum RW, et al. Protecting adolescents from harm: findings from the National Longitudinal Study on Adolescent Health. *JAMA*. 1997;278:823–832
42. Gound M, Forehand R, Long N, Miller KS, Armistead L, McNair L. Attitude mismatching: discrepancies in the sexual attitudes of African American mothers and their pre-adolescent children. *AIDS Behav*. 2007;11:113–122
43. Miller KS, Whitaker DJ. Predictors of mother-adolescent discussions about condoms: implications for providers who serve youth. *Pediatrics*. 2001;108(2). Available at: www.pediatrics.org/cgi/content/full/108/2/e28
44. Miller KS, Kotchick BA, Dorsey S, Forehand R, Ham AY. Family communication about sex: what are parents saying and are their adolescents listening? *Fam Plann Perspect*. 1998;30:218–235
45. Kahn JR, Anderson KE. Intergenerational patterns of teenage fertility. *Demography*. 1992;29:39–57
46. East PL, Felice ME. Pregnancy risk among the younger sisters of pregnant and childbearing adolescents. *J Dev Behav Pediatr*. 1992;13:128–136
47. East PL, Kiernan EA. Risks among youth who have multiple sisters who were adolescent parents. *Fam Plann Perspect*. 2001;33:75–80
48. East PL, Jacobson LJ. Mothers' differential treatment of their adolescent childbearing and nonchildbearing children: contrasts between and within families. *J Fam Psychol*. 2003;17:384–396
49. East PL, Khoo ST. Longitudinal pathways linking family factors and siblings relationship qualities to adolescent substance use and sexual risk behaviors. *J Fam Psychol*. 2005;19:571–580
50. Wilder EI, Watt TT. Risky parental behavior and adolescent sexual activity at first coitus. *Milbank Q*. 2002;80:481–524
51. Capaldi DM, Crosby L, Stoolmiller M. Predicting the timing of first sexual intercourse for at-risk adolescent males. *Child Dev*. 1996;67:344–359
52. Whitbeck LB, Simons RM, Kao M. The effects of divorced mothers' dating behaviors and sexual attitudes on the sexual attitudes and behaviors of their adolescent children. *J Marriage Fam*. 1994;56:615–621
53. Kirby D, Miller BC. Interventions designed to promote parent-teen communications about sexuality. *New Dir Child Adolesc Dev*. 2002;97:93–110
54. Robin L, Dittus P, Whitaker D, et al. Behavioral interventions to reduce incidence of HIV, STD, and pregnancy among adolescents: a decade in review. *J Adolesc Health*. 2004;34:3–26
55. Stanton BF, Li X, Galbraith J, et al. Parental underestimates of adolescent risk behavior: a randomized, controlled trial of a parental monitoring intervention. *J Adolesc Health*. 2000;26:18–26
56. Winett RA, Anderson ES, Moore JF, et al. Efficacy of a home-based human immunodefieciency virus prevention video for teens and parents. *Health Educ Q*. 1993;20:555–567
57. Blake SM, Simkin L, Ledsky R, Perkins C, Calabrese JM. Effects of a parent-child communications intervention on young adolescents' risk for early onset of sexual intercourse. *Fam Plann Perspect*. 2001;33:52–61
58. Pedlow CT, Carey MP. Developmentally appropriate sexual risk reduction interventions for adolescents: rationale, review of interventions, and recommendations for research and practice. *Ann Behav Med*. 2004;27:172–184
59. Wu Y, Stanton B, Galbraith J, et al. Sustaining and broadening intervention impact: a longitudinal randomized trial of 3 adolescent risk reduction approaches. *Pediatrics*. 2003;(1). Available at: www.pediatrics.org/cgi/content/full/111/1/e32
60. Stanton B, Cole M, Galbraith J, et al. Randomized trial of a parent intervention: parents can make a difference in long-term adolescent risk behaviors, perceptions, and knowledge. *Arch Pediatr Adolesc Med*. 2004;158:947–955

61. Mays RM, Sturm LA, Zimet GD. Parental perspectives on vaccinating children against sexually transmitted infections. *Soc Sci Med.* 2004;58:1405–1413
62. Zimet GD, Mays RM, Sturm LA, Ravert AA, Perkins SM, Juliar BE. Parental attitudes about sexually trasnsmitted infection vaccination for their adolescent children. *Arch Pediatr Adolesc Med.* 2005;159:132–137
63. Waller J, Marlow LA, Wardle J. Mothers' attitudes towards preventing cervical cancer through human papillomavirus vaccination: a qualitative study. *Cancer Epidemiol Biomarkers Prev.* 2006;15:1257–1261
64. Kahn JA, Rosenthal SL, Hamann T, Bernstein DI. Attitudes about human papillomavirus in young women. *Int J STD AIDS.* 2003;14:300–306
65. Monk BJ, Wiley DJ. Will widespread human papillomavirus prophylactic vaccination change sexual practices of adolescent and young adult women in America? *Obstet Gynecol.* 2006;108: 420–424

Religiosity, Spirituality, and Adolescent Sexuality

Sian Cotton, PhD*[a], Devon Berry, PhD[b]

[a]*Departments of Family Medicine and Pediatrics, Institute for the Study of Health, University of Cincinnati College of Medicine, PO Box 670840, Cincinnati, OH 45267-0840, USA*

[b]*University of Cincinnati College of Nursing, 3110 Vine Street, PO Box 210038, Cincinnati, OH 45221, USA*

One of the important developmental tasks for adolescents is to develop a healthy sense of sexuality, which includes feeling positive about one's body, delaying the initiation of sexual intercourse, and, if sexually experienced, engaging in health promoting behaviors such as reducing the number of sexual partners and using protective measures (ie, condoms, contraception). There are many factors that influence adolescent sexual health outcomes, including individual characteristics such as age of menarche or educational status; family characteristics such as parental monitoring or mother's openness to having conversations about sex; and sociocultural characteristics such as perceived normative behavior of peers and cultural context.[1–4] One factor that is less often considered but has individual, family, and sociocultural characteristics is religion and spirituality.

Exploring religious and spiritual factors is logical, because both have been shown to be related to reducing sexual risk and both play an important role in adolescents' lives.[5–8] Higher levels of religiosity (eg, attendance of religious services or importance of religion) in adolescents have been associated with initiating sexual intercourse later and having fewer sexual partners and less unprotected sex.[7,9,10] Adolescents who have higher levels of religiosity and spirituality fare better than their less religious or spiritual peers (they have lower rates of risky health behaviors, have fewer mental health problems, and use spiritual coping to manage physical illness) even when controlling for relevant demographic and clinical characteristics.[11–13]

Religion and spirituality indeed are important to adolescents. An estimated 84% to 95% of adolescents believe in God, 80% state that religion is important in their life (39% say "very important"), 49% say religion is very to extremely important

---

*Corresponding author.
E-mail address: sian.cotton@uc.edu (S. Cotton).

Copyright © 2007 American Academy of Pediatrics. All rights reserved. ISSN 1934-4287

in shaping major life decisions, 93% believe God loves them, 49% "definitely" believe in life after death, >50% attend religious services at least monthly and participate in religious youth groups, and close to half frequently pray alone.[6,14]

PURPOSE

The purpose of this article is to (1) define the terms "religiosity" and "spirituality," (2) synthesize the key scientific literature on the relationships among religiosity, spirituality, and adolescent sexual health outcomes (eg, coital debut, contraceptive practices), including describing why religiosity/spirituality may be related to these outcomes (ie, potential mediating pathways), and (3) discuss programs/clinical implications that incorporate these findings into improving sexual health outcomes for adolescents.

DEFINITIONS AND MEASUREMENT OF RELIGIOUS/SPIRITUAL FACTORS

Although definitions and measurement of religious and spiritual factors in research may not initially seem important to the busy practitioner, attempts to implement findings into actual practice with adolescents necessitate at least a cursory understanding of terminology. Although inconsistencies abound, religiosity and spirituality are the terms most frequently used, with "religiosity" defined as the formal, institutional, and outward expression of the sacred and "spirituality" often defined as the internal, personal, and emotional expression of the sacred.[15] Religiosity is a multidimensional construct characterized by behaviors, beliefs, values, and attitudes.[16,17] Spirituality is often defined more nebulously, incorporating a sense of connection to self, others, nature, and the divine.[15–17] Although the academic community continues to refine the definitions, measurements, and uses of the terms, adolescents themselves seem to be less concerned about these distinctions. When asked in a national survey, 8% of American teenagers said that it was very true that they are "spiritual but not religious," 46% said it was somewhat true, and 43% said it was not true of them at all[5]; however, the investigators stated that when asked that question, "most teens literally did not understand what we were asking about."[5(p78)]

It is not surprising that previous studies on this topic have used a variety of measures to assess religious/spiritual factors. By far, the most commonly used measures are that of religious attendance and denomination, as often reported in large national data sets such as the National Longitudinal Study of Adolescent Health (Add Health),[18] the National Survey of Family Growth,[19] and Monitoring the Future.[20] An exception is the National Study of Youth and Religion,[5,14] which is a nationwide random telephone survey of >3300 13- to17-year-olds and their parents conducted from 2002 to 2003. The telephone calls were followed with 267 face-to-face interviews about the role of religion and spirituality in the lives of American teenagers today and included questions about having oral sex, belief in waiting for marriage to have sex, closeness to God, and importance of religious faith in shaping daily life.[5,14] Moreover, although individual investigators often assess other domains rather than simply attendance or denomination, unfortunately their measures are often not valid for use with adolescents or developed by those investigators for the purposes of only their study, which limits their ability to generalize or draw valid conclusions.

PREVIOUS STUDIES OF RELIGIOSITY/SPIRITUALITY AND ADOLESCENT HEALTH OUTCOMES

A growing body of empirical evidence, from both adults and adolescents, supports links between religiosity, spirituality, and health outcomes, including sexual health outcomes.[12,15,21] Often described as a "protective" or "resilience" factor,[22] religiosity/spirituality has been examined in relation to several general adolescent health categories: (1) mental health (eg, depression/anxiety/suicide risk)[23]; (2) physical health (eg, research with populations of adolescents with chronic illness such as cancer or HIV)[24]; and (3) health risk behaviors (eg, drug/alcohol use, coital debut),[25] the category most often studied.[11–13] The findings presented below are those related to the sexual health topics of potentially the greatest interest to the clinician who cares for teens, including sexual behaviors and attitudes (eg, coital debut/sexual initiation, number of sexual partners) and contraception.

SEXUAL BEHAVIORS/ATTITUDES

Overall, adolescents who believe in God, rate religion as important in their lives, and attend religious services are less likely to engage in sexual intercourse at early ages; have fewer sexual partners; are less experienced sexually; and have more conservative sexual attitudes than their less religious peers.[5,7,9,10,26,27] In 2 often-cited studies by Thornton et al, those adolescents who attended church more frequently and who valued religion in their lives had the least permissive sexual attitudes (eg, "young people should not have sex before marriage") and were less experienced sexually than their less religious peers (39% of regular religious-service attenders versus 65% of rare attenders reported ever having had intercourse).[7,26] In another study, multivariate analyses of >26 000 7th- to 12th-graders (88% white and 53% male) showed that higher levels of religiosity (defined as religious feelings) was significantly associated with delayed onset of sexual activity for both boys and girls.[9] Recent analyses have shown that more religious teens less frequently endorsed other (not often studied) sexual activities such as oral sex, anal sex, and the use of Internet pornography.[5,28,29] Regarding number of sexual partners, adolescents who attended church sparingly or not at all were 6 times more likely than the most religious adolescents (24% vs 4%) to have had ≥3 sexual partners.[29] Those protective associations typically hold constant when controlling for well-established risk factors such as socioeconomic status, age at menarche, and family stability.[9,27] However, not all studies have demonstrated a significant relationship.[30,31]

It is interesting to note that the protective effects of religiosity on sexual behavior may not be present across racial subgroups and, in particular, may not be in effect in the black population.[11,28,32,33] Regnerus[28] described the following paradox: although black adolescents endorse greater importance of religion in their lives than their white peers,[20,34] they also report the highest levels of sexual involvement at an early age,[28] which is especially true for black males.[28,35] Overall, the influence of religiosity on sexual health outcomes seems strongest (ie, most protective) among white adolescent girls[11,28,35]; why this is the case, however, remains unclear. Unfortunately, we know relatively little about the influence of religion on sexual health among Latino or Asian American adolescents.[31,36]

Regarding denomination, most studies have shown that strength of religious conviction, religious salience (eg, whether religious beliefs would influence decisions about sex), and participation in religious activities (ie, services and youth groups) are more important than denominational affiliation in predicting sexual health outcomes such as abstinence or timing of sexual initiation.[26,29,33,37,38] Thornton and Camburn[7] found that religious participation was more important than specific affiliation in determining sexual attitudes and behaviors. They concluded that the content taught across major religious groups may be similarly and sufficiently opposed to sexual behavior in adolescents to merit the relatively few observed group differences. Opposing studies that have highlighted denominational differences, however, do exist.[39] Using data from the National Survey of Family Growth, Cooksey et al[40] found that white Protestant fundamentalists were much more likely to remain virgins over a 4-year time period when compared with those from other denominations. However, effects of religious affiliation or denomination are often estimated without controlling for other related factors that, when accounted for, reduce the observed denominational effects.[28]

Regarding parental influences, although adolescents' religious beliefs, traditions, and service-attendance patterns tend to reflect those of their parents,[5] few studies have assessed the relationship between parental religiosity and adolescent sexual behaviors.[28,33] Using 2 nationally representative data sets,[14,18] Regnerus[29] found that frequency of parental church attendance was inversely associated with conversations about birth control and sex but directly associated with conversations about moral issues involved in adolescent sex; that is, devoutly religious parents seemed to discuss birth control and sex less commonly with their adolescents and reported more difficulty talking about those issues. Regarding human papillomavirus vaccination acceptability, Constantine and Jerman[41] found that parents who reported no religion, who were born-again or evangelical Christians, or who were more than once-a-week religious-service attenders were less likely to endorse vaccinating their daughters before age 13 (although despite some subgroup differences, overall acceptance for the vaccine was >50%). Race differences may be present here as well. Using national longitudinal data, more frequent parental religious-service attendance was associated with delaying first intercourse among all ethnic groups except in the black population.[33]

Regarding sexual attitudes, it is not surprising that high levels of religiosity (more frequent religious-service attendance, greater importance of religion, and strong religious beliefs) have been associated with more conservative or restrictive sexual attitudes.[7,37,38] Conservative attitudes, however, do not always translate into health promoting behaviors. For example, Thornton and Camburn[7] found that although both denominational affiliation and service attendance affected attitudes about sex, only religious-service attendance affected whether adolescents actually had intercourse. More religious adolescents, especially those identified as religiously conservative, tend to anticipate or experience greater sex-related guilt and think that having sex would upset their mother (but they are less concerned what their friends will think).[28] In summary, the data support a general protective trend for higher levels of religiosity on sexual health outcomes in adolescents, although findings may differ according to dimension of religiosity assessed (public versus private religiosity; religious salience versus denomination)[42] and subgroup affiliation.[11] For example, this protective effect does not seem to hold as true for black adolescents, and the strongest observed, yet not well-understood, effect has been shown for white adolescent girls.[11,28,35]

CONTRACEPTION

Perhaps of particular interest to the practitioner who cares for teens are the data that link contraceptive practice to religious and spiritual factors in adolescents. These data have been less consistent than the overall relationships described above.[12,33] Some evidence has suggested that adolescents with higher levels of religiosity or more conservative religious affiliations may be less likely to use certain types of contraception if they do engage in sexual intercourse.[26,29,40] For example, 1 frequently cited study by Studer and Thornton[26] found that in 217 sexually experienced 18-year-olds, those who attended church regularly were more likely to use a condom, foam, cream, or jelly ("drugstore methods") and less likely to use oral contraceptive pills or intrauterine devices ("medical methods") than those who attended church less frequently. These findings were not affected by other related factors such as recent sexual activity, social class, and parents' marital stability.[26] In addition, Miller and Gur[10] reported that in 3356 adolescent girls, personal devotion to God and religious-service attendance (although not personal conservatism, defined as a rigid adherence to a religious creed) were related to greater sexual responsibility, including responsible and planned birth control use.

Still others have reported little to no relationship between religiosity (including parental religiosity) and either greater or lesser use of contraception.[27,33,42,43] In a study of 374 16- to 21-year-old Australians, sexually active, religious youth did not differ from their nonreligious peers in frequency of recent condom use, age at which they first used condoms, or rate of changing partners.[43] Using Add Health data, Nonnemaker et al[42] found that neither public religiosity (attendance of religious services and youth groups) nor private religiosity (importance of religion and frequency of prayer) were associated with birth control use at the first or most recent sexual experience.

Attitudes about contraception may also differ according to religious factors. In 1 study, very religious teens were almost twice as likely as less religious teens to say that birth control is morally wrong (11% of weekly church attenders versus 6% of those who never attend church).[29] However, that belief characterized only ~11% of the most religious youth (ie, most youth, religious or not, still think that birth control is morally acceptable).[29] In addition, when asked whether their friends would think they were "looking for sex" if they used birth control, religious differences were evident: 27% of weekly attenders versus 18% of less-than-monthly attenders agreed, as did 29% of those who said that religion was "very important" versus 14% of those who stated that religion was "not important."[29]

Similar to other sexual behaviors, there seem to be subgroup differences in contraceptive practices among adolescents. In a national sample,[33] Manlove et al[33] found that among blacks, fundamentalist Protestants were least likely to use contraception when they had sex, despite greater pill use among blacks as a whole; and among whites, Catholics and fundamentalist Protestants had lower rates of contraception use compared with other groups. They also found that in males, but not females, strong parental religious beliefs and more frequent participation in family religious activities were inversely associated with rates of contraception at first intercourse. Some experts have concluded, however, that there is little evidence that any particular religious tradition, even Catholicism, shapes contraceptive usage.[26,29]

In summary, although religious affiliation and denomination do not seem to be consistently related to contraception, religious-service attendance, in particular, does seem to be associated with contraceptive attitudes even when other variables are controlled.[29] It is concerning that more religious sexually active adolescents seem less likely to report using certain types (eg, medical methods) of contraception if they do have sex,[7,29] which then places them at risk for unintended pregnancies and sexually transmitted infections (STIs).

WHY IS RELIGIOSITY/SPIRITUALITY RELATED TO SEXUAL HEALTH OUTCOMES?

Although a clear (albeit complex) connection has been established between religious/spiritual factors and adolescent sexual behaviors/attitudes and contraceptive practices, the reasons that underlie this connection remain unclear.

Religion may act in a variety of ways to influence adolescents' sexual attitudes, decisions, and behaviors, although few reasons have been confirmed empirically.[44] One obvious way that an adolescent's religion may influence his or her sexual behavior is through prohibitions or teachings against premarital sex. Religious teachings and communicated values may affect an adolescent's belief about the appropriate timing of intercourse or the appropriateness of using contraception.[14,45] This is consistent with literature that has documented parental influence of adolescent sexual decision-making via communicated values, which indicate that adolescents whose parents discuss sexuality with them and whose parents communicate clear messages regarding their values make healthier sexual choices.[46,47]

A second way that religion may impact sexuality in adolescents is via the complex social messages and social contexts within which adolescents make sexual decisions that place them at risk for STIs and pregnancy. The socialization influence model of Wallace and Williams[48] posits that health compromising and enhancing behaviors (including sexual behaviors) emanate from a dynamic socialization process that begins in childhood and extends through adolescence. The family is the adolescent's first and primary source of socialization into norms/values about the appropriateness of sexual behavior, whereas religion, peers, and school environment operate as secondary socialization influences. Both directly and indirectly, secondary influences such as religion may affect attitudes and beliefs about contraception; what types of, if any, sexual activities are considered permissible outside of marriage; and the types of environments and relationships in which adolescents place themselves.[48]

A third plausible hypothesis is that having a deeper connection to and faith in God or the sacred may influence an adolescent to find a deeper meaning in their lives, thus indirectly promoting healthy sexual behaviors (eg, delaying sexual initiation). One proposed mediator of the religion-health connection has been meaning/sense of coherence, although the empirical evidence of this pathway is scant.[49] Other plausible pathways, described by Smith et al,[5,44] include community and leadership skills, coping skills, social/cultural capital, and extracommunity links (links to national and transnational religious organizations). It is important to recognize that these hypothesized casual pathways likely do not interact with sexual health variables as a single force but, rather, as a "combination of complex causal social processes."[5(p234)] Still others have suggested that religiosity/spirituality may impact health outcomes in a more direct manner.[50]

A few researchers have begun to test the likely indirect effects that religiosity/spirituality have on sexual health outcomes. Regnerus[28] suggested that most religious effects are, in fact, "channeled through other variables" (eg, adolescent sexual values, parent-child relations) and found that when such factors were added to his statistical regression models, they "considerably reduce the influence of the religion measures" on sexual outcomes. This makes sense logically, because it is likely not the actual attendance of church that would influence an adolescent's decisions about sex but, rather, the social network or values to which he or she is exposed at the church service that might be most influential.[28] Rostosky et al[51] found support for both direct and indirect effects of religiosity on coital debut, reporting that religiosity seemed to indirectly affect coital debut through a sexual ideology or belief system about anticipated negative consequences of engaging in sexual intercourse. Meier[38] found that the effect of religiosity on first sex diminished for both male and female adolescents when personal and relational attitudes about sex were taken into account. It is important to note that others have suggested that researchers may have the order of influence wrong, that is, adolescent sexual behavior might actually influence religiosity (although these findings have been mixed and inconclusive[5,7,28,38]); additional investigation is warranted.

PROGRAMS/CLINICAL IMPLICATIONS

The most challenging and least well-described piece of this story is how to translate these findings into actual programs and clinical interactions that could promote healthy sexuality for adolescents. In 2001, the federal government established the White House Office of Faith-Based and Community Initiatives, which allowed churches and other faith-based groups to apply for federal grants to deliver a wide range of social services (including programs for adolescents).[52,53] Although this program certainly raises issues of separation of church and state and the conundrum of promoting 1 religion over another,[53] it clearly necessitates a better understanding of how religious/spiritual factors actually influence adolescents' thoughts, decisions, and behaviors. Unfortunately, there have been relatively few rigorous evaluations of faith-based sexual education programs for adolescents (or of programs that incorporate faith) and very little written about community-religious partnerships to enhance healthy sexual development in teens.[52] Until well-designed studies that use rigorous methods test proposed mediating pathways of influence and evaluate the effectiveness of interventions, programs will continue to have little empirically based direction regarding appropriate content or implementation, which can potentially hinder their ultimate effectiveness.

Actual (non–faith-based) programmatic efforts to encourage sexual health–promoting behaviors in adolescents (ie, abstinence or delaying sexual initiation, reducing the number of partners, and using condoms/contraception) have shown mixed results.[54–56] Thus, additional resources (including those from social and community agencies such as faith-based organizations) for improving sexual health outcomes for adolescents should be studied. Some have suggested that religious institutions are an important but untapped health "ally" in our nation's effort to promote the health of our youth.[57] As such, work needs to be done to form partnerships among academic researchers, communities, and religious organizations to tackle such issues effectively. One such example of a partnership is the Columbus Congregations for Healthy Youth program, a joint faculty, pastoral, community, and Department of Public Health approach to evaluate faith-based approaches to prevent teenage pregnancy and STIs.[53] With funding from the Centers for Disease Control and Prevention and the Association of Schools of Public Health, this ongoing program's initial focus is to work with the black community and churches to evaluate faith-based approaches to teen pregnancy and STI prevention.[53]

One well-known initiative sponsored by the Southern Baptist Church has encouraged >2.5 million adolescents to take a "virginity pledge" (promising to abstain from sex until marriage); however, its results have been mixed. Bearman and Bruckner[35] evaluated the success of virginity pledging on the basis of nationally representative Add Health data and found that level of religiosity (a composite measure of frequency of prayer, church attendance, and importance of religion) and having taken a virginity pledge were related to initiating sex later even after controlling for potentially relevant covariates (eg, connectedness measures and demographics). This finding, however, was strongest in younger teens and, consistent with the race differences described above, less strong in black teens.[35] Others have posited that although most virginity pledgers seem to ultimately break their pledge, they do tend to delay having sex and have overall fewer numbers of sexual partners, which in turn reduces their lifetime exposure to STIs (despite the apparent no statistical difference in STI status during young adulthood, the fact that pledgers have had fewer sexual partners before initiating sex continues to reduce their STI-transmission risk).[29] In addition, when they do have sex, those who pledge abstinence are less likely to use birth control at first sex than those who do not pledge.[35] In contrast, another study by Rostosky et al[52] reported that taking an abstinence pledge had no additional significant effect on coital debut among a sample of virgins (who were at least 15 years old), and that male black adolescents who had either signed a virginity pledge or were more religious were significantly more likely to debut than both white non-Hispanic and black boys who were less religious and/or who had not signed a pledge. Virginity pledging as an "intervention" clearly warrants additional investigation.

CLINICAL IMPLICATIONS

In light of the findings presented above, how can an adolescent medicine practitioner use this information in discussions with adolescents and their families about healthy sexuality? It is safe to say that religious/spiritual factors are indeed related to adolescent sexual health outcomes (although why this is true remains in question).[11-13] Because much of adolescent medicine is a social and behavioral science, when adolescents' religiosity or spirituality are linked to their beliefs, motivations, cognitions, and/or perceptions, they should be asked about their religion/spirituality. For example, a practitioner might ask an adolescent how his or her religious or spiritual beliefs impact his or her sexual decision-making or decisions regarding contraception as a way to "enter into the worldview"[58] of the patient to better understand the adolescent's perspective. This way, the provider becomes a more informed and, hopefully, more effective communicator (and maybe even a better health care provider) for the patient. Even if the [religious or spiritual] beliefs are unfamiliar to the physician, are different from what the physician believes, or even conflict with the medical care plan, the purpose is to *enter into the worldview of the patient* to understand why the patient believes as she[he] does.[58]

Practically speaking, it is important to recognize that practitioners often function under intense time constraints. In addition, conversations that address religiosity or spirituality need to be culturally and developmentally appropriate, with due attention given to power dynamics within the patient-provider relationship and to acknowledging values, ethics, and boundaries typical of good patient care.[58] Concerns about the appropriate level of competency/training and comfort needed to discuss religious/spiritual issues with patients are certainly valid. An estimated 100 medical schools now incorporate spirituality into their curricula (C. Puchalski, MD, written personal communication, 2007), although approximately half of them still include the subject as an elective and rarely is there time to fully explore how to practically integrate such issues into patient care, let alone adolescent patient care.

FUTURE DIRECTIONS

Although substantive research has been conducted, many questions remain about how religiosity/spirituality actually influences adolescent sexual health outcomes. Translating findings into programs that are aimed at enhancing healthy sexuality is particularly challenging. Future studies should include (1) qualitative research with adolescents about the role of religiosity/spirituality in their sexual decision-making process, (2) quantitative research that uses advanced statistical methodologies such as structural equation modeling to test hypotheses about pathways/mechanisms of influence, (3) cross-cultural comparisons in diverse populations, that is, of non–Judeo-Christian religious backgrounds (eg, Muslims), lesbian/gay/bisexual/transgendered/questioning populations, and homeless or transient youth, and (4) examining the contextual context (eg, parents' and/or peers' religiosity/spirituality or exploring race/ethnic differences) to better delineate the social or value-based influences that operate in adolescents' development of healthy sexuality.

REFERENCES

1. Santelli J, Beilenson P. Risk factors for adolescent sexual behavior, fertility, and sexually transmitted diseases. *J Sch Health.* 1992;62:271–270
2. Kinsman S, Romer D, Fursenberg F, Schwarz D. Early sexual initiation: the role of peer norms. *Pediatrics.* 1998;102:1185–1192
3. Miller KS, Levin ML, Whitaker DJ, Xu X. Patterns of condom use among adolescents: the impact of mother-adolescent communication. *Am J Public Health.* 1998;88:1542–1544

4. Shrier L. Sexually transmitted diseases in adolescents: biologic, cognitive, psychologic, behavioral, and social issues. *Adolesc Med Clin.* 2004;15:215–234
5. Smith C, Lundquist-Denton M. *Soul Searching: The Religious and Spiritual Lives of American Teenagers.* New York, New York: Oxford University Press; 2005
6. Gallup GJ, Bezilla R. *The Religious Life of Young Americans.* Princeton, NJ: Gallup International Institute; 1992
7. Thornton A, Camburn D. Religious participation and adolescent sexual behavior and attitudes. *J Marriage Fam.* 1989;51:641–653
8. Durant RH, Sanders JM Jr, Jay S, Levinson R. Adolescent contraceptive risk-taking behavior: a social psychological model of females' use of and compliance with birth control. *Adv Adolesc Mental Health.* 1990;4:87–106
9. Lammers C, Ireland M, Resnick M, Blum R. Influences on adolescents' decision to postpone onset of sexual intercourse: a survival analysis of virginity among youths aged 13 to 18 years. *J Adolesc Health.* 2000;26:42–48
10. Miller L, Gur M. Religiousness and sexual responsibility in adolescent girls. *J Adolesc Health.* 2002;31:401–406
11. Benson PL, Donahue MJ, Erickson JA. Adolescence and religion: a review of the literature from 1970 to 1986. In: Lynn ML, Moberg DO, eds. *Research in the Social Scientific Study of Religion: A Research Annual.* Vol 1. Elsevier Science/JAI Press, US; 1989:153–181
12. Bridges LJ, Moore KA. *Religion and Spirituality in Childhood and Adolescence.* Washington, DC: Child Trends; 2002
13. Cotton S, Zebracki K, Rosenthal SL, Tsevat J, Drotar D. Religion/spirituality and adolescent health outcomes: a review. *J Adolesc Health.* 2006;38:472–480
14. Smith C. *National Study of Youth and Religion.* Available at: www.youthandreligion.org. Accessed November 7, 2007
15. Koenig HG, McCullough ME, Larson DB, eds. *Handbook of Religion and Health.* New York, NY: Oxford University Press; 2001
16. Hill PC, Pargament KI. Advances in the conceptualization and measurement of religion and spirituality: implications for physical and mental health research. *Am Psychol.* 2003;58:64–74
17. Fetzer Institute, National Institute on Aging Working Group. Multidimensional measurement of religiousness/spirituality for use in health research. Available at: www.fetzer.org/PDF/Total_Fetzer_Book.pdf. Accessed October 11, 2007
18. Udry J. *The National Longitudinal Study of Adolescent Health (Add Health), Waves I & II, 1994–1996; Wave III, 2001–2002.* Chapel Hill, NC: Carolina Population Center, University of North Carolina; 2003
19. Centers for Disease Control and Prevention. National Survey of Family Growth. Available at: www.cdc.gov/nchs/nsfg.htm. Accessed May 29, 2007
20. Johnston L, Bachmna J, O'Malley P. *Monitoring the Future: Questionnaire Responses From the Nation's High School Seniors.* Ann Arbor, MI: Institute for Social Research; 1999
21. Ellison CG, Levin JS. The religion-health connection: evidence, theory, and future directions. *Health Educ Behav.* 1998;25:700–720
22. Masten ASR, Marie-Gabrielle J. Resilience in development. In: Snyder CR, Lopez SJ, eds. *Handbook of Positive Psychology.* New York, NY: Oxford University Press; 2002:74–88
23. Wong YJ, Rew L, Slaikeu KD. A systematic review of recent research on adolescent religiosity/spirituality and mental health. *Issues Ment Health Nurs.* 2006;27:161–183
24. Pendleton SM, Cavalli KS, Pargament KI, Nasr SZ. Religious/spiritual coping in childhood cystic fibrosis: a qualitative study. *Pediatrics.* 2002;109(1). Available at: www.pediatrics.org/cgi/content/full/109/1/e8
25. Cotton S, Larkin E, Hoopes A, Cromer BA, Rosenthal SL. The impact of adolescent spirituality on depressive symptoms and health risk behaviors. *J Adolesc Health.* 2005;36:529.e7–529.e14
26. Studer M, Thornton A. Adolescent religiosity and contraceptive usage. *J Marriage Fam.* 1987;49:117–128
27. Zelnik M, Kantner J, Ford K. *Sex and Pregnancy in Adolescence.* Beverly Hills, CA: Sage; 1981

28. Regnerus M. Religion and adolescent sexual behavior. In: Ellison C, Hummer R, eds. *Religion, Families, and Health.* New Brunswick, NJ: Rutgers University Press; 2008: In press
29. Regnerus M. *Forbidden Fruit: Sex and Religion in the Lives of American Teenagers.* New York, NY: Oxford University Press; 2007
30. Kellinger KG. Factors in adolescent contraceptive use. *Nurse Pract.* 1985;10:55–62
31. Villarruel A. Cultural influences on the sexual attitudes, beliefs, and norms of Latina adolescents. *J Soc Pediatr Nurs.* 1998;3:69–79; quiz 80–81
32. Benson PL, Donahue MJ. Ten-year trends in at-risk behaviors: a national study of black adolescents. *J Adolesc Res.* 1989;4:125–139
33. Manlove JS, Terry-Humen E, Ikramullah EN, Moore KA. The role of parent religiosity in teens' transitions to sex and contraception. *J Adolesc Health.* 2006;39:578–587
34. Donahue MJ. Religion and the well-being of adolescents. *J Soc Issues.* 1995;51:145–160
35. Bearman P, Bruckner H. Promising the future: virginity pledges and first intercourse. *Am J Soc.* 2001;106:859–912
36. Regnerus M, Smith C, Fritsch M. *Religion in the Lives of American Adolescents: A Review of the Literature.* Chapel Hill, NC: University of North Carolina; 2003
37. Sheeran P, Abrams D, Abraham C, Spears R. Religiosity and adolescents' premarital sexual attitudes and behaviour: an empirical study of conceptual issues. *Eur J Soc Psychol.* 1993;23: 39–52
38. Meier A. Adolescents' transition to first intercourse, religiosity, and attitudes about sex. *Soc Forces.* 2003;81:1031–1052
39. Sheeran P, Spears R, Abraham SCS, Abrams D. Religiosity, gender, and the double standard. *J Psychol.* 1996;130:23–33
40. Cooksey EC, Rindfuss RR, Guilkey DK. The initiation of adolescent sexual and contraceptive behavior during changing times. *J Health Soc Behav.* 1996;37:59–74
41. Constantine N, Jerman P. Acceptance of human papillomavirus vaccination among Californian parents of daughters: a representative statewide analysis. *J Adolesc Health.* 2007;40:108–115
42. Nonnemaker JM, McNeely CA, Blum RW. Public and private domains of religiosity and adolescent health risk behaviors: evidence from the National Longitudinal Study of Adolescent Health. *Soc Sci Med.* 2003;57:2049–2054
43. Dunne MP, Edwards R, Lucke J, Donald M, Raphael B. Religiosity, sexual intercourse and condom use among university students. *Aust J Public Health.* 1994;18:339–341
44. Smith C. Theorizing religious effects among American adolescents. *J Sci Study Relig.* 2003;42: 17–30
45. Frank NC, Kendall SJ. Religion, risk prevention and health promotion in adolescents: a community-based approach. *Ment Health Relig Cult.* 2001;4:133–148
46. Whitaker DJ, Miller KS, May DC, Levin ML. Teenage partners' communication about sexual risk and condom use: the importance of parent-teenager discussions. *Fam Plann Perspect.* 1999;31:117–121
47. Miller K, Whitaker D. Predictors of mother-adolescent discussions about condoms: implications for providers who serve youth. *Pediatrics.* 2001;108(2). Available at: www.pediatrics.org/cgi/content/full/108/2/e28
48. Wallace JM, Williams DR. Religion and adolescent health-compromising behavior. In: Schulenberg J, Maggs JL, eds. *Health Risks and Developmental Transitions During Adolescence.* New York, New York: Cambridge University Press; 1997:444–468
49. George LK, Ellison CG, Larson DB. Explaining the relationships between religious involvement and health. *Psychol Inq.* 2002;13:190–200
50. Fabricatore A, Handal P, Rubio D, Gilner F. Stress, religion and mental health: religious coping in mediating and moderating roles. *Int J Psychol Relig.* 2004;14:91–108
51. Rostosky SS, Regnerus MD, Wright ML. Coital debut: the role of religiosity and sex attitudes in the Add Health Survey. *J Sex Res.* 2003;40:358–367
52. Steinman KJ, Wright V, Cooksey E, Myers LJ, Price-Spratlen T, Ryles R. Collaborative research in a faith-based setting: Columbus Congregations for Healthy Youth. *Public Health Rep.* 2005;120:213–216

53. Glazer S. *Faith-Based Initiatives*. 2001 Congressional Quarterly Press. Available at: www.cqpress.com/product/Researcher-Faith-Based-Initiatives.html. Accessed November 7, 2007
54. Ahern NR, Kiehl EM. Adolescent sexual health & practice: a review of the literature—implications for healthcare providers, educators, and policy makers. *Fam Community Health*. 2006;29:299–313
55. Johnson B, Carey M, Marsh K, Levin K, Scott-Sheldon L. Interventions to reduce sexual risk for the human immunodeficiency virus in adolescents, 1985–2000. *Arch Pediatr Adolesc Med*. 2003;157:381–388
56. Robin L, Dittus P, Whitaker D, et al. Behavioral interventions to reduce incidence of HIV, STD, and pregnancy among adolescents: a decade in review. *J Adolesc Health*. 2004;34:3–26
57. Wallace JM, Forman TA. Religion's role in promoting health and reducing risk among American youth. *Health Educ Behav*. 1998;25:721–741
58. Koenig H. *Spirituality in Patient Care: Why, How, When, and What*. Radnor, PA: Templeton Foundation Press; 2002

From Calvin Klein to Paris Hilton and MySpace: Adolescents, Sex, and the Media

Jane D. Brown, PhD[a], Victor C. Strasburger, MD[*,b]

[a]School of Journalism and Mass Communication, University of North Carolina, 360 Carroll Hall CB 3365, Chapel Hill, NC 27599-3365, USA

[b]Department of Pediatrics, University of New Mexico School of Medicine, MSC10 5590, Albuquerque, New Mexico 87131, USA

In the absence of widespread, effective sex education at home or school, the media have become one of the leading sources of sexual information and norms in the United States today (see Fig 1).[1] Calvin Klein's sexual sell, Paris Hilton's sexual exhibitionism, and adolescents' sexual representations of themselves on social networking sites such as MySpace have made the media the arbiter of what is hot and what is not (see Fig 2). As 1 group of researchers put it: "Long before many parents begin to discuss sex with their children, answers to such questions as 'When is it OK to have sex?' and 'With whom does one have sexual relations?' are provided by messages delivered on television."[1,2] The problem is that the media rarely provide sexually healthy messages, so the sexual worldview young people get is one in which sex is glamorous, fun, and risk free.

ADOLESCENTS' USE OF MEDIA

Adolescents in the United States today have unprecedented access to an array of media, including television [TV], movies, music, magazines, and the Internet. A majority of adolescents have a TV in their own bedrooms, and most spend much more time with the media than they spend with their parents or in school. According to nationally representative surveys of 8- to 18-year-olds in 1998 and 2004, media use is equivalent to a full-time job, because, on average, adolescents spend >40 hours/week with some form of media.[3,4] High-speed Internet access, cell phones with video screens, and portable music devices such as iPods have made media use a 24/7 behavior for many. Much of the content to which they attend includes messages and images about sexual attraction, romantic relation-

---

*Corresponding author.
E-mail address: VStrasburger@salud.unm.edu (V. C. Strasburger).
Portions of this article will appear in the chapter "Sex and the Media" in the second edition of *Children, Adolescents, & the Media*, which will be published by Sage in 2008.

Copyright © 2007 American Academy of Pediatrics. All rights reserved. ISSN 1934-4287

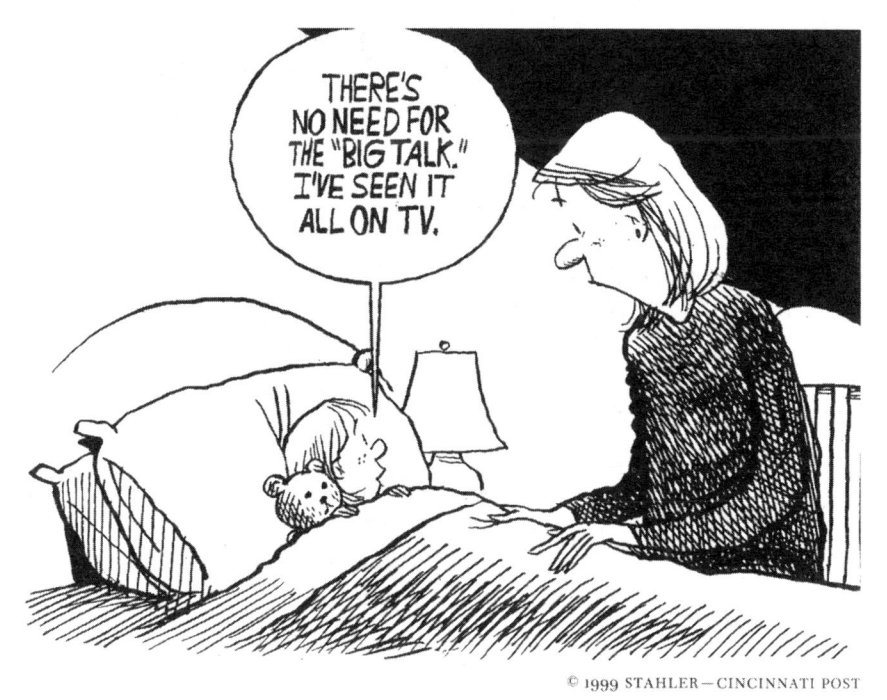

Fig 1. Source: Jeff Stahler; reprinted by permission of Newspaper Enterprise Association, Inc.

ships, and sexual behavior. Very little of this content includes any information about sexual health.

SEXUAL CONTENT IN THE MEDIA

Television

More than three fourths of prime-time shows on the major networks contain sexual content, but only 14% of sexual incidents include any mention of the risks or responsibilities of sexual activity or the need for contraception (see Fig 3).[5] Talk about sex or sexual behavior can occur as often as 8 to 10 times per hour of prime-time TV.[6] Since the 1997–1998 TV season, the amount of sexual content has nearly doubled, but there has been little change in responsible content. In the top 15 to 20 shows watched by adolescents, nearly half (45%) to two thirds contain sexual talk or behavior, with intercourse depicted or implied in 10% of the programs.[5–7] Only 10% of the top 20 teen shows mention any of the responsibilities or risks (eg, waiting to have sex, using contraception, the possibility of pregnancy or sexually transmitted diseases [STDs]) that go with having sex. Only 1% of all the shows with sexual content include precaution, prevention, or negative outcomes as the primary theme. Movies and situation comedies contain the most sexual content of all programming on TV.[5]

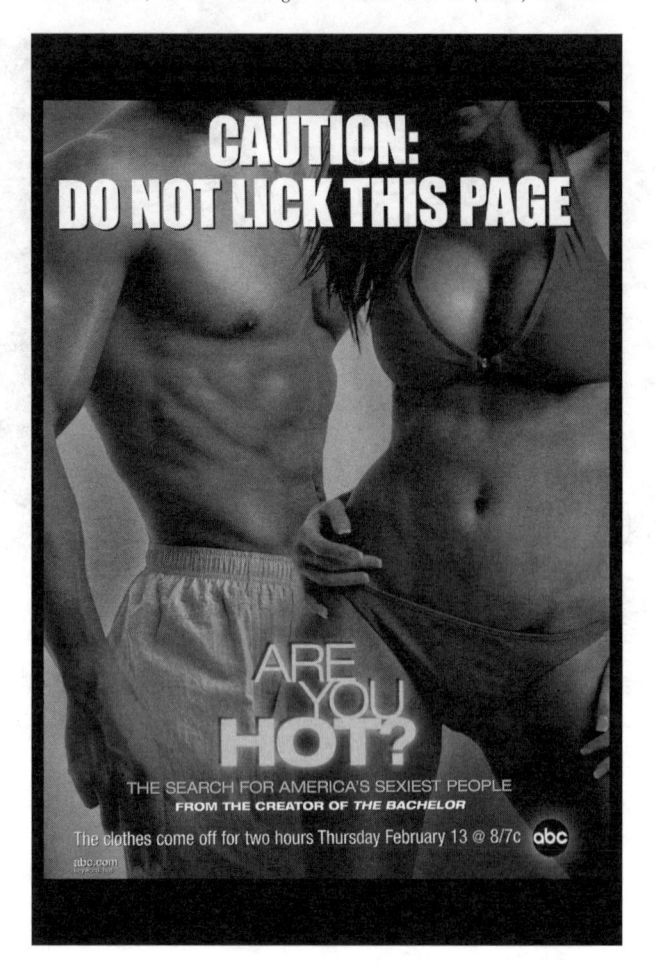

Fig 2.

Heterosexuality still prevails in mainstream TV content. Estimates of characters in TV programming who are gay, lesbian, or bisexual vary from 1.3% to 15%.[8,9] In addition, the double standard is alive and well: in an analysis of sex portrayed in prime-time shows that feature adolescents, female sexual activity was more likely to have negative consequences than male sexual activity.[10] The most frequently occurring messages depict sexual relations as a competition in which men comment on women's physical appearance and masculinity is equated with being sexual.[11,12]

What is shown on American TV is largely unrealistic, suggestive sexual innuendo or unhealthy sexual behavior.[1,13] It is sex as a casual pastime, a romp in the hay, with few or no consequences. These depictions about sex and sexual behavior on TV contrast dramatically with the fact that in the new millennium,

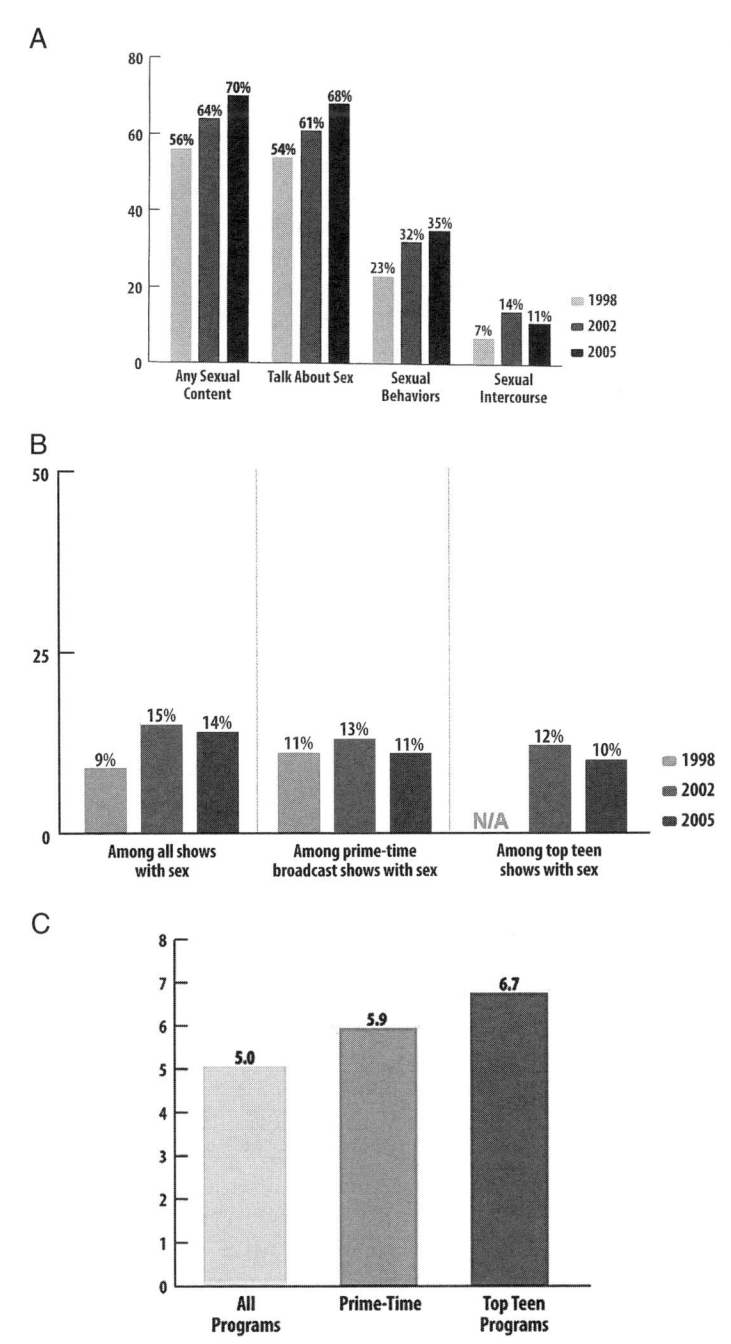

Fig 3. A, Percentages of shows with sexual content over time according to type of content. B, Percentages that also included references to risks or responsibilities over time for all shows with sexual content. C, Numbers of sex-related scenes per hour for shows in 2005 with sexual content. Reprinted courtesy of Kaiser Family Foundation.

adolescent sexuality and sexual activity (teen pregnancy, AIDS, other STDs, and abortion) have all become battlegrounds in the public health and political arenas.

Reality TV

Despite its name, reality TV is anything but real.[14,15] Nevertheless, this subterfuge genre grew immensely popular in the early 2000s. Five of the top 20 shows in the Nielsen ratings for June 26 through July 2, 2006, for example, were reality shows.[16] Sexually oriented shows are the most common type of reality TV shows and vary from all-out voyeurism ("Real World," and "Are You Hot?") to dating shows such as "The Bachelorette" and MTV's "Parental Control." In 1997, there were only 3 reality dating shows; by 2004, there were >30.[17] Some shows such as "Temptation Island" and "Paradise Hotel" bring participants together for the sole purpose of seeing who "hooks up." In a study of college students, viewing reality dating shows was correlated with beliefs in a double standard: that men are sex-driven and that men and women are sexual adversaries.[17] It is interesting to note that the less sexually experienced students were most likely to be watching more of the reality dating shows, which suggests the importance of such programs for sexual socialization.

Soap Operas

Nine hours of network soap operas daily attract >40 million viewers in the United States, and the audience is not limited to Americans. The soap opera "The Bold and the Beautiful" is the most watched TV show in the world, with an estimated 300 million viewers in 110 countries.[18] Soap operas rival reality shows in representing the most sensational and inaccurate view of adolescent and adult sexuality.

As with prime-time programming, soap operas have become even more sexually oriented and sexually explicit since the 1980s. An analysis of 10 episodes of each of the 5 top-rated soap operas ("General Hospital," "All My Children," "One Life to Live," "The Young and the Restless," and "Days of Our Lives") in 1994 found an average of 6.6 sexual incidents per hour.[19] Sex was visually depicted twice as often as it was talked about. Nearly half of the sexual incidents involved intercourse, usually between unmarried partners. It is surprising that rape was the second-most frequently depicted sexual activity, with a total of 71 incidents or 1.4 per hour. Of the 333 sexual incidents, contraception or "safe sex" was mentioned only 5 times. The only mention of AIDS among the 50 episodes concerned the risk associated with intravenous drug use, not sex, and there was only 1 episode in which a mother discussed sex with her teenage daughter. By the 1996 season, the amount of sexual content had stabilized at ~6 sexual incidents per hour, but as with prime-time shows, there seemed to be a shift from talking about sex to showing more sexual behavior. Only 10% of sexual episodes involved the use of contraception or discussions about the risks of sexual activity.[20]

However, soap-opera producers have also been more responsive to national health issues than prime-time producers.[20,21] In the 1990s, several soap operas began to run major story lines with significant health-related content: "General Hospital" (ABC) was the first to feature a character with HIV, who at one point discussed with her partner the need to use condoms if they had intercourse. On "The Young and the Restless" (CBS), a woman got tested for HIV after learning about her husband's affairs.

Magazines

Many teenagers, especially girls, rely on magazines as an important source of information about sex, birth control, and health-related issues.[22,23] A content analysis of British magazines for teens found that girls' magazines tend to focus on romance, emotions, and female responsibility for contraception, whereas boys' magazines are more visually suggestive and assume that all males are heterosexual.[24] Earlier analyses of *Seventeen* and *Sassy* found that most of the stories in these 2 teen-girl magazines contained very traditional socialization messages, including that girls depend on someone else to solve their personal problems, that girls are obsessed with boys, and that girls are appearance-conscious shoppers.[25] According to sociologist Jean Kilbourne,[26] magazines give adolescent girls impossibly contradictory messages: be innocent but be sexually experienced, too. Older teen-girl magazines such as *Jane* are filled with articles such as "How Smart Girls Flirt," "Sex to Write Home About," "15 Ways Sex Makes You Prettier," and "Are You Good in Bed?" *Sassy* initially featured more empowering and sexually responsible content such as "Losing Your Virginity" and "My Girlfriend Got Pregnant" and included a condom in an ad. However, after an advertising boycott organized by the religious right, such content was withdrawn, and the magazine ultimately folded.[27]

Magazines, in general, are more likely to discuss contraception and advertise birth control products than TV is.[28] A content analysis of teen magazines found that they devoted an average of 2 pages per issue to sexual issues. Of sexual articles in teen magazines, nearly half (42%) concerned health issues.[29] The October 2005 issue of *Seventeen*, for example, featured a frank, 2-page discussion of gynecological health entitled "Vagina 101," which won a Maggie Award from the Planned Parenthood Federation of America.[30] Much of the health coverage in teen magazines is in the form of advice columns, however, and the overarching focus seems to be on decision-making about when to lose one's virginity.[29]

Music

Popular music has always focused on love and sex and generated criticism for the sexual connotations of both the music and lyrics. As rock and roll entered the scene in the early 1950s, criticism and outrage was levied at the "throbbing sexual implications of rock's rough, primitive, musical structure and the provocative physical gyrations these 'jungle rhythms' produced in performers and audience alike."[31(p116)]

Although the music itself continues to evoke visceral response and objection, primarily from adults, most criticism and research has focused on the lyrics and visual images now associated with the music through music videos. Debate continues about whether young listeners actually know the words and/or interpret lyrics as sexual, but lyrics are much more accessible now than ever before. Most CDs include a full transcript of the words, and various Web sites feature lyrics to most of the songs ever recorded. An analysis of the lyrics on albums to which early adolescents (12- to 14-year-olds) listened most frequently in 2002 revealed that music included the most references to sex of any of the 4 media (music, movies, magazines, and TV) studied. Overall, 40% of the lyric lines made some reference to bodies as sexual objects, relationships, and/or intercourse.[32] Only ~6% of the lyric lines included any mention of what might be construed as sexually healthy messages (eg, physical/sexual development, refusal of advance/ abstinence, masturbation, STDs, negative emotional consequences, condoms, and contraception).

There has been little behavioral research on the impact of music lyrics and music videos. However, 1 recent study did find an association between listening to music with "sexually degrading lyrics" and earlier onset of sexual intercourse and other sexual activity.[33]

Pornography/Sexually Explicit Media

The Internet has been a key factor in increasing access to sexually explicit content. In the late 1990s, it was estimated that the online pornography industry was worth $1 billion and that half of all spending on the Internet was related to sexual activity. Content includes not only conventional material such as online versions of *Playboy* but also hardcore magazines that previously have been available only in X-rated bookstores or by mail. The Internet also provides space for discussion and depiction of unconventional and bizarre sexual interests (eg, discussion groups on almost any sexual paraphilia), as well as pornographic picture libraries, live strip and sex shows, and voyeuristic Web-cam sites.[34] In all of these genres, "the pursuit of sexual access is typically presented as relentless and exploitative (the object is to score), that sex is a sporting event that amounts to innocent fun, and that it is inconsequential for subsequent emotions and health."[35]

Teens may sometimes have more trouble avoiding sexual material online than they have accessing it. In a 2001 study, 70% of 15- to 17-year-olds in the United States reported that they had "accidentally" seen pornography on the Internet.[36]

In another survey, about one fourth of 10- to 17-year-olds said they had experienced unwanted exposure to pictures of naked people or people having sex while online.[37] Two years after that, Ybarra and Mitchell[38] concluded from a nationally representative youth Internet-safety survey of 1500 youths aged 10 to 17 that nearly all (95%) teens who accessed pornography online were male, and most were >14 years old, an age at which sexual curiosity is developmentally appropriate. They concluded that concerns about large numbers of healthy, well-adjusted adolescents being exposed to online pornography were overstated. Research on pre-Internet pornography seems to have supported that conclusion (as long as violence is not involved).[1]

Although concerns about youth access to online pornography have waned slightly, a new concern has taken center stage in the new millennium: the creation of online sexual content by teens. With the growth of user-generated content in chat rooms and on bulletin boards, personal home pages, blogs, and, most recently, social networking sites, adolescents have had greater opportunity than ever before to present themselves publicly to a geographically disparate audience. Many young people choose to post pictures of themselves in poses and clothes that could be considered sensual and sexually suggestive. Some also write about their sexual identities, sexual behaviors, and sexual desires online. For example, Stern[39] found that, among the 233 teen home pages she analyzed, nearly one tenth of the authors mentioned sex, with girls 3 times as likely as boys to do so.

The possibility that teens' own sexual content might invite sexual predation by adults (usually men) has led to substantial apprehension. Concerns also surround the idea that the provocative and/or sexual imagery that teens, especially girls, post online is a form of self-objectification in which young people "learn to think of and treat their own bodies as objects of others' desires." In so doing, young people may "internalize an observer's perspective on their physical selves and learn to treat themselves as objects to be looked at and evaluated for their appearance."[40]

Advertising

From the time of the Noxema girl, who advised male viewers to "take it off, take it all off," to Brooke Shields' "Nothing comes between me and my Calvins" to present-day ads for beer, wine coolers, and perfume, advertising has always used explicit visual imagery to try to make a sale.[26] Teenaged girls spend an estimated $25 billion per year on cosmetics alone.[41] Even in the 1980s, a study of 4000 network commercials found that 1 of every 3.8 ads relied on attractiveness-based imagery.[42] A study of >1750 commercials in TV shows watched by early adolescents (12- to 14-year-olds) in 2001 found that the commercials often contained more sexual content than the surrounding programs. Most of the sexual imagery focused on the body and sexual touching between unmarried couples.[43]

In magazine ads, women are as likely to be shown in suggestive clothing (30%), partially clad (13%), or nude (6%) as they are to be fully clothed.[44] Although research on the sexual objectification of men is scarce, male bodies are increasingly being portrayed in more sexually explicit ways, essentially becoming "more masculinized" by revealing muscled, "buff" bodies.[45]

Advertisers seem to be wrestling with how to portray both sexes. One TV car ad, for example, showed 2 women discussing whether men buy big cars because they are worried about the size of their penises: "He must be overcompensating for a...shortcoming?" says one. Then a handsome man drives up in a Hyundai Elantra, and her friend says, "I wonder what he's got under the hood."[46] On the flip side, ads for erectile dysfunction (ED) drugs are ubiquitous. In the first 10 months of 2004, the makers of ED drugs spent $343 million on advertising.[47] Mentions of "4-hour erections" are not uncommon, even on programs with primarily young audiences.[1]

Modern advertising often features women's bodies that have been "dismembered" (only the legs or breasts appear), and even little girls are sexualized (eg, a shampoo ad reads, "You're a Halston woman from the very beginning" and shows a girl of ~5 years old).[26] A study of fashion and fitness ads in popular magazines found that females are more likely than males to be shown in submissive positions, sexually displayed, or to be included in violent imagery.[48] As Kilbourne noted, "When sexual jokes are used to sell everything from rice to roach-killer, from cars to carpets, it is hard to remember that sex can unite two souls, can inspire awe. Individually, these ads are harmless enough, sometimes even funny, but the cumulative effect is to degrade and devalue sex."[26]

LEARNING ABOUT SEX FROM THE MEDIA

Content analyses can determine what kind of sexual norms are current in the media, but they do not reveal what teenagers actually learn from these portrayals. Apart from their pervasiveness, accessibility, and sexualized content, the media may be powerful sex educators primarily because other sources of information and norms are absent, silent, or punitive. In the context of a culture that provides little information about sexuality through conventional socialization channels such as parents, schools, and religion but condones a media environment replete with sexual content, the media have become important sexual socialization agents. Sex-education programs may increasingly be "abstinence only," but the media are decidedly not.

Adolescents frequently cite the media as sources of sexual information.[49] Because friends and even parents may also be influenced by what they see, hear, and read in the media about sex, the cumulative effects of the media may outweigh other influences. In a 2004 national survey of 519 teens aged 15 to 19, the media far outranked parents or schools as a source of information about birth control.[50]

A growing number of studies have documented the media's ability to transmit information about sex, shape attitudes and perceptions of sexual norms, and encourage sexual activity.[1,51,52] Most of the research has focused on the effects of TV as an especially powerful medium, because it combines visuals and audio and is watched for 3 to 4 hours every day by most young Americans. TV influences viewers' perception of social behavior and social reality,[53] contributes to the development of cultural norms,[54] and offers teenagers "scripts" for sexual behavior that they might not be able to observe elsewhere.[55]

The Media's Influence on Sexual Norms and Scripts

Surveys and experiments have found that the media do influence teens' ideas about what is sexually "normal" and how people should act in sexual situations. In 1 experiment, for example, older adolescents who saw TV shows that depicted sexual relationships rated casual sex less negatively than those who did not view the programs.[56] Other studies have found that frequent soap-opera viewers are more likely than those who watch less to have unrealistic notions about the ease of single motherhood,[57] and teens who watch talk shows frequently are more likely to believe that the unusual sexual behavior presented on talk shows is realistic.[58] One national survey found that 40% of teenagers said that they had learned ideas about how to talk with their boyfriends or girlfriends about sex directly from media portrayals.[59]

Researchers have also examined the impact of sexual content on attitude formation. For example, adolescents who viewed only 10 music videos were more likely to agree with the notion that "premarital sex is acceptable,"[60] and college students who were shown sexually explicit films reported a greater acceptance of sexual infidelity and promiscuity than did controls.[61] College students' disapproval of rape was lessened by viewing sexually explicit films,[62] and both males and females reported less satisfaction with their intimate partners.[63]

The media may function as a kind of "super-peer" that encourages teens to have sex earlier than they might otherwise.[64,65] Several studies have documented that teens who are avid consumers of media are more likely to overestimate the number of their peers and friends who are sexually active and to feel more pressure from the media to begin having sex than from friends.[49] Three fourths of the 13- to 19-year-olds who responded to an anonymous *Seventeen* survey believed that most teenagers are having sex, whereas only about half actually are.[66] Greater exposure to sexual content on TV is correlated with higher expectations of the sexual activity of peers and a more positive attitude toward recreational sex.[67] Heavy doses of TV may accentuate teens' feelings that everyone is "doing it" except them and may contribute to their desire to have sex, too.

The Media's Effects on Teens' Sexual Behavior

In the 1990s, after 40 years of research on media violence and aggressive behavior, researchers began focusing on whether the media might also be a cause of earlier sexual activity. With encouragement from Congress, the National Institutes of Health issued a call for proposals to investigate the effects of the media on adolescents' sexual behavior. A number of large-scale longitudinal studies were funded, and some of the initial findings are now available. Such studies take us closer to establishing the causal sequence of the media's effects, because they measure adolescents' media use and sexual behavior over time and in the teen's natural setting.

Collins et al,[68] in a National Institutes of Health–funded longitudinal study of a nationally representative sample of 12- to 17-year-olds, concluded that early exposure to sexual content on TV "hastens" initiation of sexual intercourse, on average, by ~6 months. Similar findings were reported from data from the National Longitudinal Study of Adolescent Health. In an analysis of nearly 5000 teenagers aged <16 years who had not yet had sexual intercourse, researchers found that those who watched >2 hours of TV per day were nearly twice as likely to begin having sex within 1 year compared with lighter viewers.[69] Brown et al,[70] in a longitudinal study in North Carolina, found that early adolescents who had heavier sexual media diets across 4 media (music, movies, TV, and magazines) were twice as likely as those with lighter sexual media diets to have initiated sexual intercourse by the time they were 16 years old. The relationship was stronger for white than black adolescents after controlling for other factors that could affect either exposure to the media and/or sexual behavior, including closeness to parents and perceptions of peers' sexual behavior (see Figs 4 and 5). These studies suggest that the media do contribute to adolescents' early initiation of sexual intercourse.

Differences in Media Use and Interpretation

Although Collins et al[68] found that exposure to sex on TV predicted earlier sexual intercourse for both black and white adolescents, Brown et al[70] found that for black teens the strength of the link between media exposure at 12 to 14 years and sexual behavior 2 years later disappeared when perceptions of parental expectations and peers' sexual behavior were taken into account. They speculated that the effect of the media may occur earlier for black children both because black children, on average, can mature earlier and the media to which black teens attend is more sexual than the media that white teens typically use.[70]

As we learn more about the media's role in adolescents' sexual socialization, it is increasingly clear that this is a complicated process in which selection, attention, interpretation, and sometimes even resistance to media content as well as other contexts are important factors. Social-demographic identities, such as

Proportion of Adolescents Reporting Sexual Intercourse by Age and Sexual Media Diet

Teen Media researchers calculated each teen's Sexual Media Diet (SMD) by combining the sexual content in the media teens used with the amount of time they spent using each type of media. White teens with a high SMD were 2.2 times more likely to have had sexual intercourse two years later than White teens with a low SMD. The increase in sexual intercourse for Blacks was not statistically significant.

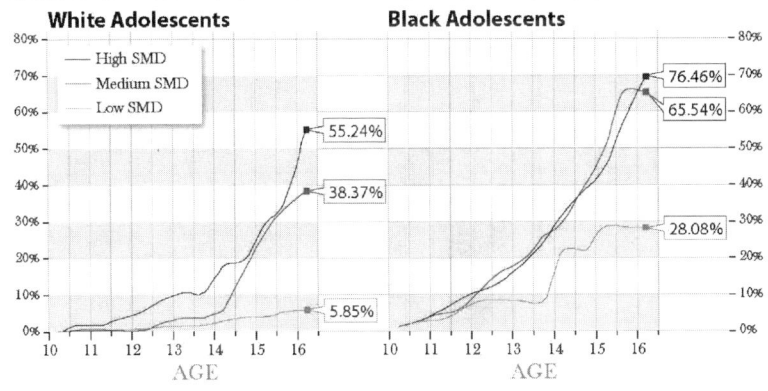

Fig 4.

gender and race/ethnicity, as well as personality characteristics and other socialization contexts, affect which media are selected, to which content teens pay attention, and to what extent it is incorporated into a teen's everyday life and sense of sexual self.[71]

Media use and effects do not occur in isolation and are affected by the teen's family configuration and interactions (eg, do older siblings choose what's on? Does the family have rules about content exposure and/or time spent with media?) as well as peers (eg, do friends use and discuss the same media?). Additional study of these and other potential mediators and moderators of the relationship between media exposure and teen sexual behavior is necessary in both theoretical understanding of the process of media effects and designing media interventions for sexual health.

One of the core developmental tasks of adolescence is developing a sense of self in relation to others and the culture. Gender and race/ethnicity are 2 key components of identity that affect both which media content is chosen and how it is interpreted. The digital revolution has resulted in an amazing array of channels of TV, movies, and music that will soon all be available on computers and portable devices. From very early on, it has been as if boys and girls live in different media worlds, because girls tend to choose more relationship-oriented content and boys choose sports and action-adventure.[72] Boys are much more likely to attend to pornography on the Internet than girls,[73] which matters because boys and girls may be getting very different views of sexuality in the content they choose.

Race also affects media selection, use, and interpretation. In 1 study of teens' TV

How much, if at all, do you think the sexual behaviors on TV influence the sexual behaviors of teens your age?

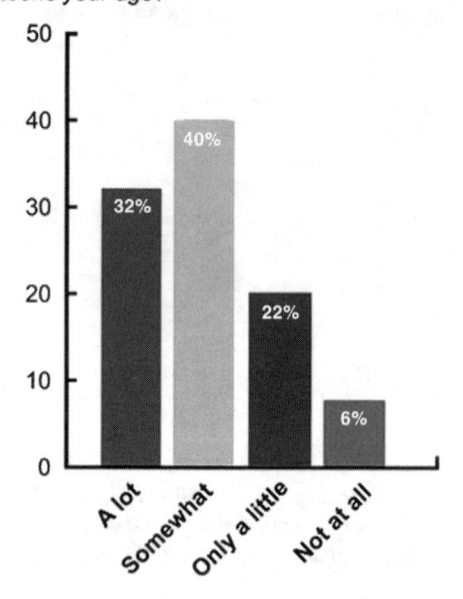

- A lot: 32%
- Somewhat: 40%
- Only a little: 22%
- Not at all: 6%

How much, if at all, do you think the sexual behaviors on TV influence your own sexual behavior?

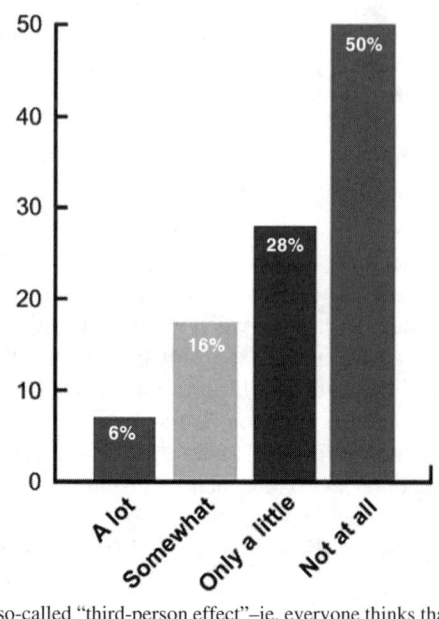

- A lot: 6%
- Somewhat: 16%
- Only a little: 28%
- Not at all: 50%

Fig 5. An example of the so-called "third-person effect"–ie, everyone thinks that the media influences other people, but not themselves. Reprinted courtesy of Kaiser Family Foundation.

use, black and white and male and female adolescents had only 4 of a list of 150 current TV shows in common. The majority of black teens, both boys and girls, regularly watched shows that featured black casts, whereas white girls and boys rarely watched shows with black casts and tended to choose gender-stereotypical fare.[74] In 2002, for example, the TV show with the largest number of teen-girl viewers was "American Idol," a show that chose a new singing star from amateur contenders. Teen boys, meanwhile, were watching "World Wrestling Entertainment" and National Football League games.[75]

Another example of race and gender differences in interpretation is a study of older adolescents' reactions to Madonna's video "Papa Don't Preach."[76] Black male teens viewed the popular music video as a father-daughter-boyfriend story rather than a story about teen pregnancy, apparently because they identified more with the plight of the boyfriend, and the young woman Madonna played did not appear physically pregnant. Most of the girls who saw it, however, focused on the girls' predicament and interpreted the lyrics, "Papa, I'm in trouble deep," as meaning that she was pregnant.

THE POTENTIAL OF MEDIA INTERVENTIONS FOR SEXUAL HEALTH

The media have been used effectively to promote sexual and reproductive health in other countries for decades.[77] The media may be especially useful for teaching young people about sexual and reproductive health practices for precisely the same reasons that they are influential in promoting sexually risky behaviors. Teens may find the media to be a less embarrassing way to learn about sex than talking with a parent or other adult, and messages can be presented in the media that teens use frequently by media characters they admire and wish to emulate. A few media-based campaigns in the United States have suggested that the media could be used in the promotion of sexual health and pregnancy prevention. Few of these have been set up as field experiments or evaluated systematically, however, which is what is needed now.

Four kinds of media-based interventions are worth pursuing: contraceptive advertising, sexual health media campaigns, entertainment-education, and media-literacy education.

Contraceptive Advertising

In 1976, the NBC Standards and Practices Department (the network's censors) refused to allow writer Dan Wakefield use the word "responsible" when "James at 15" and his girlfriend were about to have sexual intercourse for the first time and wanted to discuss birth control.[78] To date, the networks still reject public service announcements (PSAs) and ads about contraception in fear that they will offend some unknown but vocal population in America's hinterland.[1] Meanwhile, ads for Viagra, Cialis, and Levitra are abundant and make sex seem like a recreational sport. If an occasional ad for a birth control product does make it to the air, it is presented because of the noncontraceptive properties of the product (eg, Ortho Tri-Cyclen is usually advertised as a treatment for acne, not a means of preventing pregnancy).

For years, a large majority of adults have supported the airing of information about HIV and AIDS prevention and favored condoms being discussed and/or advertised on TV.[79] It certainly seems odd, perhaps even hypocritical, that as the culture has become increasingly "sexualized" in the past 20 years, the 1 taboo remaining is the public mention of birth control. The apparent "disconnect" between the networks' willingness to air ads for ED drugs and their unwillingness to air ads for birth control products seems hypocritical at best.[80]

Would advertising of condoms and birth control pills have an impact on the rates of teen pregnancy or acquisition of HIV? International studies have suggested that such advertising could help. When Zaire began advertising condoms, condom sales increased 20-fold in only 3 years (from 900 000 in 1988 to 18 million in 1991).[81] Would advertising birth control products make teenagers more sexually active than they already are? There has been no evidence to indicate that allowing freer access to birth control encourages teenagers to become sexually active at a younger age. In fact, at least 8 studies have suggested the opposite; giving teens freer access to condoms does not increase their sexual activity or push virginal teenagers into having sex but does increase the use of condoms among those who are sexually active.[82] Organizations such as the American Academy of Pediatrics, the American College of Obstetricians and Gynecologists, and the Society for Adolescent Medicine have all called for contraceptive advertising on American TV.[13]

Sexual Health Media Campaigns

In 2002, MTV and Advocates for Youth sponsored a year-long campaign focused on HIV/AIDS, other STDs, and unintended pregnancy. The campaign included special programming, public service messages, and a comprehensive sexual health Web site for youth. A survey in 2003 of MTV viewers (16–24 years old) found that of those who had seen the campaign, three fourths were more likely to take a relationship seriously and to use a condom if they had sex. Two thirds of the respondents said they were more likely to talk to a boyfriend or girlfriend about safer sex and to wait to have sex.[83]

On a more local level, an intensive 3-year effort in 1 county in New York that included TV and radio ads and an interactive Web site, as well as schools and peer educators, resulted in significant drops in early teen sexual intercourse and pregnancy in comparison with the surrounding counties.[84] The mass media have also been used proactively to try to increase parent-child communication about sex. In North Carolina, a mass media campaign used billboards and radio and TV PSAs with the theme of, "Talk to your kids about sex. Everyone else is." The impact of the campaign was assessed via a postexposure survey given to 1132 parents of adolescents who lived in the 32 counties covered by the campaign. Exposure to a billboard message or PSA significantly correlated with a parent talking to their children about sex during the following month.[85]

From evaluations of other sexual health-related media interventions such as these, it is clear that to be effective, media campaigns must reach target audiences with clear messages and be sustained over time. Stimulation of interpersonal communication and access to health services also would increase desired outcomes.[86]

Entertainment-Education

Embedding sexual health messages in entertainment programming has been found to be especially effective at persuading audiences to seek and use contraceptives, to limit the size of their families, and to postpone sexual behavior in a number of countries around the world.[77] The advantage of entertainment-education over traditional media campaigns is that the complexity that surrounds sexual issues (relationships, values, love, parents, regret) can be explored in entertainment media in much more depth and with more nuance and less preachiness than the typical PSA.

In the United States, the technique also has been effective but more limited, given the difficulty of working with a highly commercialized media free from government control. Two groups (the National Campaign to Prevent Teen Pregnancy and, in partnership with the Kaiser Family Foundation, the Advocates for Youth–sponsored Media Project) have been most effective in working with the entertainment media to get responsible sexual health messages in media content that adolescents and/or their parents see.

Since the late 1990s, the National Campaign to Prevent Teen Pregnancy has generated pregnancy prevention-related programming that has reached >300 million teens and parents on all 6 TV networks and top cable outlets, in national magazines, and on leading Web sites. The campaign encouraged media producers to explore the motivations behind adolescents' decisions to either wait to have sex or use protection if they do have sex and to get teens to engage in conversation about their own decision-making. Entertainment media already tailored to different teen-audience segments (eg, younger girls, urban teens) were used to approach these issues in ways that are most relevant to the targeted teen-audience segment.

Those who created the campaign also developed innovative ways of increasing the teen audience's involvement with the material. After 1 episode of a show and a PSA that promoted the campaign's Web site, viewers were encouraged to answer questions that challenged them to relate what happened in the show to their own lives. The campaign researchers then shared the responses with other teens and with network executives so they could see the kind of response that a show about teen sex, relationships, and pregnancy engendered in their audience. They learned that regular viewers care a lot about what their favorite characters do, and when these super-peers begin dealing with sex and pregnancy, viewers react and talk about it.

Rigorous evaluation of the effectiveness of such efforts has been sparse but promising. During the 1999 TV season, the Media Project worked with the producers of "Felicity" on a 2-part episode about date rape. The project encouraged the creation of a toll-free rape crisis hotline number to be displayed at the end of the episode, and the hotline received >1000 calls directly after the show aired.[87] In a small survey about a later episode that discussed birth control, more than one fourth of the 12- to 21-year-olds surveyed felt that they had learned something new about birth control and safe sex. Another evaluation found that exposure to a 3-minute discussion on the TV program "ER" increased viewers' awareness of emergency contraception 17 percentage points, and a 1-minute discussion of human papilloma virus increased viewers' awareness 23 percentage points. The show also stimulated viewers to talk with friends and family about the topics.[88] A study of adolescent viewers of a "Friends" episode in which a pregnancy resulted from condom failure found that up to two thirds of them learned that condoms can fail, and another one third learned about condoms' efficacy in preventing pregnancy.[89] An experiment with college students found that young women who saw episodes of popular TV shows with depictions of condoms held more favorable attitudes toward condoms than women who saw shows that depicted sexual intercourse but no condoms.[90]

In 2003, media giant Viacom and the Kaiser Family Foundation launched an ambitious project to produce $120 million worth of PSAs and print ads concerning HIV/AIDS and encourage Viacom producers to include storylines in their TV shows that would raise AIDS awareness (see Fig 6).[91] Such efforts demonstrate that the entertainment industry can be remarkably receptive to outside input and that healthier content can be introduced into mainstream TV without government pressure or the threat of censorship.

Media-Literacy Education

Another promising strategy is media-literacy education. Media-literacy education typically focuses on increasing awareness of how media are produced and packaged. It is a relatively new approach to helping young people make good decisions about their health. The assumption is that adolescents will become more critical of what they see and hear and will be less likely to engage in the unhealthy behavior promoted in the media. Although media-literacy education has been practiced in other countries such as Canada, Great Britain, and Australia

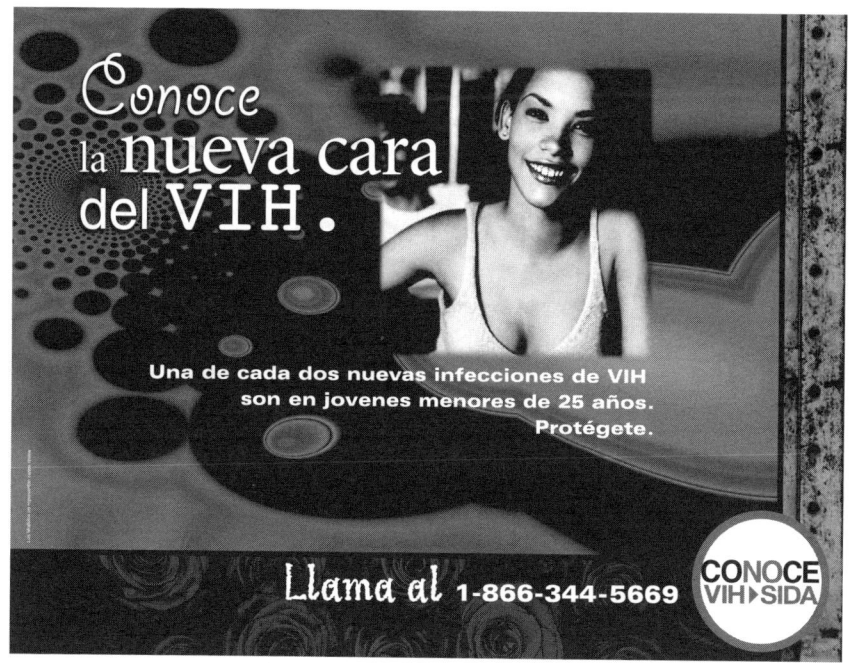

Fig 6.

for ≥3 decades, it is just now gaining a foothold in the United States. The movement has spawned 2 national organizations that advance media-education training, networking, and information exchange through professional conferences and media Listservs: Alliance for a Media Literate America and Action Coalition for Media Education.

In 1997 the American Academy of Pediatrics launched a national "Media Matters" media-education campaign designed to educate its members and provide clinical tools to assess and mitigate media effects on children and adolescents. The kit included a "media history" form that pediatricians were encouraged to have parents fill out to assess their children's patterns of media use. Apparently, only a few pediatricians used the form, because they found it to be too time-consuming. Pediatrician researcher Michael Rich surveyed US pediatric residency programs and found that only about one third of them teach about the health effects of media exposure. He concluded that "developing a pediatric media curriculum and training pediatric residency directors or designated faculty may be a resource-effective means of improving health for children growing up in a media-saturated environment."[92]

The media-literacy movement in the United States has been hampered, however, by a lack of rigorous evaluations of the various media-literacy interventions that are underway.[93] Only a few previous studies have established that media-literacy training increases critical thinking about the media and/or affects attitudes about health issues[94] (eg, alcohol and tobacco use, body image, and violence). It is not clear at this point how much media education is necessary, when it should start, how long it should last, or what components are most important. Most existing media-education curricula require multiple meetings and focus on only 1 medium (usually TV and/or advertising) or only 1 health issue at a time.

One recent study, however, showed that even 1 media-literacy training session can increase early adolescents' skepticism toward advertising and that taking a more emotional rather than only a fact-based approach may be most effective for children in middle school.[95] Another study found that the greater the knowledge about the persuasion techniques of cigarette advertising, the less likely teens were to smoke cigarettes.[96] Media-literacy interventions focused on the norms of sexual behavior presented in the media may be helpful with reducing the effect of the media's portrayals on adolescents.

CONCLUSIONS

Even in the new millenium, researchers continue to fight the old shibboleth that if you ask kids about sex, they will get ideas they would otherwise not have had.[1] Although half of high school seniors have had sexual intercourse, and adolescents are bombarded with sexual messages in the media, school administrators and parents are still reluctant to have teenagers questioned about their sexual activities, even with the use of informed consent. In addition, the federal government and private foundations have been reluctant to fund any sort of media research, much less research on sex and the media. Hence, only a few large-scale studies of the impact of the media on adolescents' sexual behavior have been conducted. Clearly, that needs to change, but so does the uniquely American attitude that teaching about sex and sexuality is harmful. Numerous government studies have shown that abstinence-only sex education is not effective.[97] Because the media are not abstinence only, sex-education programs cannot afford to be; they must be proactive in dealing with a wide variety of sexual issues and they must be comprehensive, especially in dealing with contraception.

Programming needs to change as well. Censorship is not desirable, but the entertainment industry needs to understand that it has a public health responsibility. Casual, suggestive, unhealthy sexuality, particularly in programming that might be viewed by children or adolescents, is not appropriate. The mention of risks and responsibilities needs to increase from 10%–14% of all sexual references to at least a majority. Pro-social messages can be embedded easily in shows that are popular with teenagers without interfering with anyone's First Amendment rights. Although the Internet is an attractive target, the public needs to understand that it is essentially unregulatable,[98] because the only possible solution, addition of a ".xxx" domain to isolate pornography, has not been widely accepted.

Finally, parents and pediatricians need to stop being "clueless" about the media's impact on young people.[65] Two brief questions in a well-child or well-teen visit could be extremely useful: "How much screen media time do you spend, per day, for entertainment?" and "Is there a TV set (and Internet connection) in your bedroom?" Parents, too, seem reluctant to try to control their youngsters' media access or choices despite the recommendations of the American Academy of Pediatrics and the research that shows its importance.

Parents have long been clueless about their teenagers' activities,[99] but media seem to rank around 63 on a list of things about which parents want to think. That needs to change. Current research is clear: the media may have a significant impact on virtually every concern that parents and pediatricians have about young people—sex, drugs, aggressive behavior, academic success, obesity, eating disorders, and even suicide. In the new millennium, parents and pediatricians will have to discontinue their traditional "ostrich" approach to dealing with media effects and become far more proactive if teenagers are to thrive in a media-saturated environment.

REFERENCES

1. Strasburger VC. Adolescents, sex, and the media: ooooo, baby, baby: a Q & A. *Adolesc Med Clin.* 2005;16:269–288, vii
2. Kunkel D, Cope KM, Biely E. Sexual messages on television: comparing findings from three studies. *J Sex Res.* 1999;36:230–236
3. Roberts DF, Foehr UG. *Kids and Media in America.* Cambridge, United Kingdom: Cambridge University Press; 2004
4. Rideout V, Roberts DF, Foehr UG. *Generation M: Media in the Lives of 8–18 Year-Olds.* Menlo Park, CA: Kaiser Family Foundation; 2005
5. Kunkel D, Eyal K, Finnerty K, Biely E, Donnerstein E. *Sex on TV 4: A Biennial Report to the Kaiser Family Foundation.* Menlo Park, CA: Kaiser Family Foundation; 2005
6. Kunkel D, Cope KM, Colvin C. *Sexual Messages on Family Hour Television: Content and Context.* Menlo Park, CA: Kaiser Family Foundation; 1996
7. Cope-Farrar KM, Kunkel D. Sexual messages in teens' favorite prime-time TV programs. In: Brown JD, Steele JR, Walsh-Childers K, eds. *Sexual Teens, Sexual Media.* Hillsdale, NJ: Lawrence Erlbaum; 2002:59–78
8. Fisher DA, Hill DL, Grube JW, Grube EL. Sex on American television: an analysis across program genres and network types. *J Broadcast Electronic Media.* 2004;48:529–553
9. Moore F. Study: fewer gay television characters. Available at: http://abcnews.go.com/Entertainment/print?id=2340204. Accessed August 22, 2006
10. Aubrey JS. Sex and punishment: an examination of sexual consequences and the sexual double standard in teen programming. *Sex Roles.* 2004;50:505–514
11. Strasburger VC. Risky business: what primary care practitioners need to know about the influence of the media on adolescents. *Prim Care.* 2006;33:317–348
12. Ward LM. Talking about sex: common themes about sexuality in the prime-time television programs children and adolescents view most. *J Youth Adolesc.* 1995;24:595–615
13. American Academy of Pediatrics, Committee on Public Education; American Psychological Association. Sexuality, contraception, and the media. *Pediatrics.* 2001;107:191–194

14. Hill A. *Reality TV: Audiences and Popular Factual Television*. Oxford, United Kingdom: Routledge; 2005
15. Murray S, Ouellette L, eds. *Reality TV: Remaking Television Culture*. New York, NY: NYU Press; 2005
16. Nielsen ratings, June 26–July 2. Available at: http://www.accessmylibrary.com/coms2/summary_0286-16296732_ITM. Accessed July 6, 2006
17. Zurbriggen EL, Morgan EM. Who wants to marry a millionaire? Reality dating television programs, attitudes toward sex, and sexual behaviors. *Sex Roles*. 2006;54:1–17
18. Stern BB, Russell CA, Russell DW. Vulnerable women on screen and at home: soap opera consumption. *J Macromark*. 2005;25:222–225
19. Greenberg BS, Busselle RW. *Soap Operas and Sexual Activity*. Menlo Park, CA: Kaiser Family Foundation; 1994
20. Heintz-Knowles KE. *Sexual Activity on Daytime Soap Operas: A Content Analysis of Five Weeks of Television Programming*. Menlo Park, CA: Kaiser Family Foundation; 1996
21. Centers for Disease Control and Prevention Sentinel for Health Award: writers and producers gather to address the role of women in daytime dramas. Available at: http://www.population.org/summits/soapsummit/cdcaward.htm. Accessed May 25, 2007
22. Treise D, Gotthoffer A. Stuff you couldn't ask your parents about: teens talking about using magazines for sex information. In: Brown JD, Steele JR, Walsh-Childers K, eds. *Sexual Teens, Sexual Media*. Mahwah, NJ: Lawrence Erlbaum; 2002: 173–189
23. Wray J, Steele J. Girls in print: figuring out what it means to be a girl. In: Brown JD, Steele JR, Walsh-Childers K, eds. *Sexual Teens, Sexual Media*. Mahwah, NJ: Lawrence Erlbaum; 2002: 191–208
24. Batchelor SA, Kitzinger J, Burtney E. Representing young people's sexuality in the "youth" media. *Health Educ Res*. 2004;19:669–676
25. Peirce K. Socialization of teenage girls through teen-magazine fiction: the making of a new woman or an old lady? *Sex Roles*. 1993;29:59–68
26. Kilbourne J. *Deadly Persuasion: Why Women and Girls Must Fight the Addictive Power of Advertising*. New York, NY: Free Press; 1999
27. Brown JD, Steele JR. *Sex and the Mass Media*. Menlo Park, CA: Kaiser Family Foundation; 1995
28. Walsh-Childers K, Gotthoffer A, Lepre CR. From "just the facts" to "downright salacious:" teens' and women's magazines' coverage of sex and sexual health. In: Brown JD, Steele JR, Walsh-Childers K, eds. *Sexual Teens, Sexual Media*. Mahwah, NJ: Lawrence Erlbaum; 2002: 153–171
29. Walsh-Childers K. *A Content Analysis: Sexual Health Coverage in Women's, Men's, Teen and Other Specialty Magazines*. Menlo Park, CA: Kaiser Family Foundation; 1997
30. Planned Parenthood Federation of America. PPFA Maggie Awards. Available at: www.plannedparenthood.org/news-articles-press/politics-policy-issues/ppfa-maggie-awards-10047.htm. Accessed May 25, 2007
31. Christenson PG, Roberts DF. *It's Not Only Rock & Roll: Popular Music in the Lives of Adolescents*. Cresskill, NJ: Hampton Press; 2001
32. Pardun CJ, L'Engle K, Brown JD. Linking exposure to outcomes: early adolescents' consumption of sexual content in six media. *Mass Commun Soc*. 2005;8:75–91
33. Martino SC, Collins RL, Elliott MN, Strachman A, Kanouse DE, Berry SH. Exposure to degrading versus nondegrading music lyrics and sexual behavior among youth. *Pediatrics*. 2006;118(2). Available at: www.pediatrics.org/cgi/content/full/118/2/e430
34. Griffiths M. Sex on the Internet: issues, concerns and implications. In: Von Feilitzen C, Carlsson U, eds. *Children in the New Media Landscape: Games, Pornography, Perceptions*. Gotenborg, Sweden: UNESCO Clearinghouse on Children and Violence on the Screen; 2000:169–184
35. Zillmann D. Influence of unrestrained access to erotica on adolescents' and young adults' dispositions toward sexuality. *J Adolesc Health*. 2000;27(2 suppl):41–44
36. Rideout V. *Generation RX.com: How Young People Use the Internet for Health Information*. Menlo Park, CA: Kaiser Family Foundation; 2000

37. Mitchell KJ, Finkelhor D, Wolak J. The exposure of youth to unwanted sexual material on the Internet: a national survey of risk, impact, and prevention. *Youth Soc.* 2003;34:330–358
38. Ybarra ML, Mitchell KJ. Exposure to Internet pornography among children and adolescents: a national survey. *Cyberpsychol Behav.* 2005;8:473–486
39. Stern S. Sexual selves on the World Wide Web: adolescent girls' home pages as sites for sexual self-expression. In: Brown JD, Steele JR, Walsh-Childers K, eds. *Sexual Teens, Sexual Media.* Mahwah, NJ: Lawrence Erlbaum; 2002:265–286
40. American Psychological Association. Report of the APA Task Force on the Sexualization of Girls. Available at: www.apa.org/pi/wpo/sexualizationsum.html. Accessed May 25, 2007
41. Rowe J. Grossly distorting perception. Available at: www.theecologist.org/archive_detail.asp?content_id=400. Accessed May 25, 2007
42. Downs AC, Harrison SK. Embarrassing age spots or just plain ugly? Physical attractiveness stereotyping as an instrument of sexism on American television commercials. *Sex Roles.* 2003;13:9–19
43. Pardun CJ, Forde KR. Sexual content of television commercials watched by early adolescents. In: Reichert T, Lambiase J, eds. *Sex in Promotional Culture: The Erotic Content of Media and Marketing.* Mahwah, NJ: Lawrence Erlbaum; 2006:125–139
44. Reichert T, Carpenter C. An update on sex in magazine advertising: 1983 to 2003. *Journal Mass Commun Q.* 2004;81:823–837
45. Reichert T, Lambiase J, Morgan S, Carstarphen M, Zavoina S. Cheesecake and beefcake: no matter how you slice it, sexual explicitness in advertising continues to increase. *Journal Mass Commun Q.* 1999;76:7–20
46. Leo J. '90s advertisements portray women with "attitude." *Albuquerque Journal.* October 20, 1993:A11
47. Snowbeck C. FDA tells Levitra to cool it with ad. Available at: www.post-gazette.com/pg/05109/490334.stm. Accessed July 20, 2005
48. Rudman WJ, Verdi P. Exploitation: comparing sexual and violent imagery of females and males in advertising. *Women Health.* 1993;20(4):1–14
49. Kaiser Family Foundation/Children Now. *The Family Hour Focus Groups: Children's Responses to Sexual Content on TV and Their Parents' Reactions.* Menlo Park, CA: Kaiser Family Foundation; 1996
50. Kaiser Family Foundation/Seventeen Magazine. *Sex Smarts: Birth Control and Protection.* Menlo Park, CA: Kaiser Family Foundation; 2004
51. Escobar-Chaves SL, Tortolero S, Markham C, Low B. *Impact of the Media on Adolescent Sexual Attitudes and Behaviors.* Austin, TX: Medical Institute for Sexual Health; 2004
52. Ward LM. Understanding the role of entertainment media in the sexual socialization of American youth: a review of empirical research. *Dev Rev.* 2003;33:347–388
53. Bandura A. *Social Learning Theory.* Englewood Cliffs, NJ: Prentice Hall; 1993
54. Gerbner G, Gross L, Morgan M, Signorielli N, Shanahan J. Growing up with television: cultivation processes. In: Bryant J, Zillmann D, eds. *Media Effects: Advances in Theory and Research.* 2nd ed. Hillsdale, NJ: Lawrence Erlbaum; 2002:43–68
55. Gagnon JH, Simon W. The sexual scripting of oral genital contacts. *Arch Sex Behav.* 1987;16:1–25
56. Bryant J, Rockwell SC. Effects of massive exposure to sexually-oriented primetime television programming on adolescents' moral judgment. In: Zillmann D, Bryant J, Huston AC, eds. *Media, Children, and the Family: Social Scientific, Psychodynamic, and Clinical Perspectives.* Hillsdale, NJ: Lawrence Erlbaum; 1994:183–195
57. Larson MS. Sex roles and soap operas: what adolescents learn about single motherhood. *Sex Roles.* 1996;35:97–110
58. Greenberg BS, Smith SW. Daytime talk shows: up close and in your face. In: Brown JD, Steele JR, Walsh-Childers K, eds. *Sexual Teens, Sexual Media.* Hillsdale, NJ: Lawrence Erlbaum; 2002:79–93

59. Kaiser Family Foundation. *Kaiser Family Foundation and YM Magazine National Survey of Teens: Teens Talk About Dating, Intimacy, and Their Sexual Experiences.* Menlo Park, CA: Kaiser Family Foundation; 1998
60. Greeson LE, Williams RA. Social implications of music videos for youth: an analysis of the contents and effects of MTV. *Youth Soc.* 1986;18:177–189
61. Zillmann D. Erotica and family values. In: Zillmann D, Bryant J, Huston AC, eds. *Media, Children, and the Family: Social Scientific, Psychodynamic, and Clinical Perspectives.* Hillsdale, NJ: Lawrence Erlbaum; 1994:19–213
62. Zillmann D, Bryant J. Pornography, sexual callousness and the trivialization of rape. *J Commun.* 1982;32:10–21
63. Zillmann D, Bryant J. Pornography's impact on sexual satisfaction. *J Appl Soc Psychol.* 1988;18:438–453
64. Brown JD, Halpern CT, L'Engle KL. Mass media as a sexual super peer for early maturing girls. *J Adolesc Health.* 2005;36:420–427
65. Strasburger V. "Clueless:" why do pediatricians underestimate the media's influence on children and adolescents? *Pediatrics.* 2006;117:1427–1431
66. Tucker K. Kids these days. *Entertainment Weekly.* December 17, 1999:62–63
67. Ward LM, Gorvine B, Cytron A. Would that really happen? Adolescents' perceptions of sexual relationships according to prime-time television. In: Brown JD, Steele JR, Walsh-Childers K, eds. *Sexual Teens, Sexual Media.* Hillsdale, NJ: Lawrence Erlbaum; 2002:95–123
68. Collins RL, Elliott MN, Berry SH, et al. Watching sex on television predicts adolescent initiation of sexual behavior. *Pediatrics.* 2004;114(3). Available at: www.pediatrics.org/cgi/content/full/114/3/e280
69. Ashby SL, Arcari CM, Edmonson MB. Television viewing and risk of sexual initiation by young adolescents. *Arch Pediatr Adolesc Med.* 2006;160:375–380
70. Brown JD, L'Engle K, Pardun CJ, Guo G, Kenneavy K, Jackson C. Sexy media matter: exposure to sexual content in music, movies, television, and magazines predicts black and white adolescents' sexual behavior. *Pediatrics.* 2006;117:1018–1027
71. Steele JR, Brown JD. Adolescent room culture: studying media in the context of everyday life. *J Youth Adolesc.* 1995;24:551–576
72. Hust SJ, Brown JD. Gender, media use and effects. In: Calvert SL, Wilson BJ, eds. *Blackwell Handbook of Child Development and the Media.* New York, NY: Blackwell; 2008: In press
73. Peter J, Valkenburg PM. Adolescents' exposure to sexually explicit material on the Internet. *Commun Res.* 2006;33:178–204
74. Brown JD, Pardun CJ. Little in common: racial and gender differences in adolescents' TV diets. *J Broadcast Electronic Media.* 2004;48:266–278
75. *Teen Media Monitor.* Menlo Park, CA; Kaiser Family Foundation; 2003
76. Brown JD, Schulze L. The effects of race, gender, and fandom on audience interpretations of Madonna's music videos. *J Commun.* 1990;40:88–102
77. Singhal A, Rogers EM. *Entertainment-Education: A Communication Strategy for Social Change.* Mahwah, NJ: Lawrence Erlbaum; 1999
78. Wakefield D. Teen sex and TV: how the medium has grown up. *TV Guide.* November 7, 1987:4–6
79. Kaiser Family Foundation. Public and networks getting comfortable with condom advertising on TV [press release]. Menlo Park, CA: Kaiser Family Foundation; June 19, 2001
80. Strasburger VC; American Academy of Pediatrics, Committee on Communications. Children, adolescents, and advertising [published correction appears in *Pediatrics.* 2007;119:424]. *Pediatrics.* 2006;118:2563–2569
81. Alter J. The power to change what's "cool." *Newsweek.* January 17, 1994:23
82. Kirby D, Brener ND, Brown NL, Peterfreund N, Hillard P, Harrist R. The impact of condom distribution in Seattle schools on sexual behavior and condom use. *Am J Public Health.* 1999;89:182–187
83. Kaiser Family Foundation. *National Survey of Teens and Young Adults on Sexual Health Public Education Campaigns: Topline Results.* Menlo Park, CA: Kaiser Family Foundation; 2003

84. Doniger AS, Adams E, Utter CA, Riley JS. Impact evaluation of the "Not Me, Not Now" abstinence-oriented adolescent pregnancy prevention communications program, Monroe County, New York. *J Health Commun.* 2001;6:45–60
85. DuRant RH, Wolfson M, LaFrance B, Balkrishnan R, Altman D. An evaluation of a mass media campaign to encourage parents of adolescents to talk to their children about sex. *J Adolesc Health.* 2006;38:298.e1–298.e9
86. Wellings K. Evaluating AIDS public education in Europe: a cross-national comparison. In: Hornik RC, ed. *Public Health Communication: Evidence of Behavior Change.* Mahway NJ: Lawrence Erlbaum; 2002:131–146
87. Folb KL. "Don't touch that dial!" TV as a—what!?—positive influence. *SIECUS Rep.* 2000;28: 16–18
88. Brodie M, Foehr U, Rideout V, et al. Communicating health information through the entertainment media. *Health Aff (Millwood).* 2001;20:1–8
89. Collins RL, Elliott MN, Berry SH, Kanouse E, Hunter SB. Entertainment television as a healthy sex educator: the impact of condom-efficacy information in an episode of Friends. *Pediatrics.* 2003;112:1115–1121
90. Farrar KM. Sexual intercourse on television: do safe sex messages matter? *J Broadcast Electronic Media.* 2006;50:635–650
91. Tannen T. Media giant and foundation team up to fight HIV/AIDS. *Lancet.* 2003;361:1440–1441
92. Rich M, Bar-on M. Child health in the information age: media education of pediatricians. *Pediatrics.* 2001;107:156–162
93. Kubey R. Obstacles to the development of media education in the United States. *J Commun.* 1998;Winter:58–69
94. McCannon R. Media literacy/media education: solution to big media? In: Strasburger VC, Wilson BJ, Jordan A, eds. *Children, Adolescents, & the Media.* Thousand Oaks, CA: Sage; 2008: In press
95. Austin EA, Chen YC, Pinkleton BE, Johnson JQ. Benefits and costs of *Channel One* in a middle school setting and the role of media-literacy training. *Pediatrics.* 2006;117(3). Available at: www.pediatrics.org/cgi/content/full/117/3/e423
96. Primack, BA, Gold MA, Land SR, Fine MJ. Association of cigarette smoking and media literacy about smoking among adolescents. *J Adolesc Health.* 2006;39:465–472
97. Trenholm C, Devaney B, Fortson K, Quay L, Wheeler J, Clark M. *Impacts of Four Title V, Section 510 Abstinence Education Programs: Final Report.* Princeton, NJ: Mathematica Policy Research; 2007
98. Donnerstein E. The Internet. In: Strasburger VC, Wilson BJ, Jordan A, eds. *Children, Adolescents, & the Media.* Thousand Oaks, CA: Sage; 2008: In press
99. Young TL, Zimmerman R. Clueless: parental knowledge of risk behaviors of middle school students. *Arch Pediatr Adolesc Med.* 1998;152:1137–1139

Adolescent Sexual Orientation

Michael G. Spigarelli, MD, PhD*

Division of Adolescent Medicine, Cincinnati Children's Hospital Medical Center, 3333 Burnet Avenue, Cincinnati, OH 45229, USA

Sexual orientation has been defined as the patterns of sexual thoughts, fantasies, and attractions that an individual has toward other persons of the same or opposite gender. Although it can be defined, it is rarely understood as defined. In reality, as most concur, sexual orientation can be a very difficult issue to fully grasp, whether it applies to themselves, their family members, their patients, or anyone else. Most societies, both historical and modern, have a tendency to view sexual orientation solely as a choice; thus, they cannot adequately deal with any differences or ambiguities from the presumed "norm." This inability to deal with differences, especially when discussing sexuality, tends to increase the complexity of the topic. With respect to sexual orientation, "normal" tends to be viewed as the predominant cultural ideal; thus, the depth and breadth of diverse thoughts and experiences that contribute to adolescent and adult sexual orientation cannot be fully embraced.

Despite the fact that same-sex relationships have been recorded throughout history, the terms "homosexual" and "heterosexual" were conceived relatively recently, with the first recorded use between 1869 and 1892.[1] In 1974, the American Academy of Psychiatry removed homosexuality from the list of mental illnesses, choosing to view it as an alternative of sexual expression.[2] In the medical and scientific literature, it is understood that sexual orientation is not chosen. In fact, there have been studies that demonstrated an association between sexual orientation and brain structures, which provides supporting evidence that sexual orientation is not a choice but an intrinsic characteristic of each individual. The first of these studies to make the case for an observable biological difference showed that an area of the third interstitial nucleus of the anterior hypothalamus was smaller in both heterosexual females and homosexual males.[3] Several other studies have demonstrated neuroanatomic dimorphisms between heterosexual and homosexual males, although there has not been a demonstration of sexual orientation dimorphisms in females.[4] Additional evidence for a biological basis for sexual orientation can be seen with 2 putative human pheromones; one was

---

*Corresponding author.
E-mail address: spig@cchmc.org (M. G. Spigarelli).

Copyright © 2007 American Academy of Pediatrics. All rights reserved. ISSN 1934-4287

found in male sweat and another was found in female urine. Maximal activation of the medial preoptic area/anterior hypothalamus, which in animals is highly associated with sexual behaviors, is observed in heterosexual males when exposed to the female-produced compound. This same type of activation was also seen in heterosexual females and homosexual males to the putative male pheromone.[5]

Regardless of the biological or social components, it does take time for sexual orientation to become fully apparent and to be recognized and accepted by the individual and then by others. Throughout childhood and approaching adolescence, children try to understand their own sexuality and sexual orientation in the context of the society in which they live. Typically, this attempt to understand first occurs in thoughts of a sexual nature and later through actions, usually before sexual orientation is clearly defined. How these experiences are handled, by the individual and close friends and relatives, helps to define how an individual views and accepts their sexual orientation ultimately as an adult. The level of difficulty that each individual encounters serves as the basis for the observed increased rates of risk behaviors such as substance abuse and suicidal ideation.

Individuals who are not part of the sexual majority or are uncertain of their sexual orientation are referred to as lesbian, gay, bisexual, transgender, or questioning (LGBTQ). This article is intended to provide information about the development of sexual identity in an effort to improve the comfort level of providers who interact with adolescents.

DEVELOPMENT OF SEXUAL IDENTITY

Adolescent sexual identity formation passes through several stages, with distinct phases from initial sexual thoughts through actions such as sexual intercourse, which has been well detailed and is beyond the scope of this article.[6] This process takes place within a myriad of other transitions for adolescents and is more complicated for youth in the sexual minority. These transitions can be a source for concern to adolescents and their family, friends, and health care providers, yet they are not frequently discussed in either the home or health care settings. This discomfort stems from many sources, including include lack of knowledge of the subject matter and fear of discovering sexual behavior is occurring, which will then require other uncomfortable (for the provider) interventions or discussions. In addition, providers sometimes worry that asking about behaviors may inadvertently condone them and will experience anxiety about damaging the relationship with the parents or patient, among numerous other unfounded fears. Parents and providers may worry about the societal consequences for anyone in the sexual minority and desire to protect their child from scrutiny or pressure.

Although adolescents in the sexual minority face many of the same issues that all racial, ethnic, or religious minorities encounter, there are specific differences. Adolescents and young adults who self-identify as LGBTQ are typically raised within heterosexual households. When they face discrimination or prejudice outside their home because of their orientation, it limits the level of coping mechanisms that can be discussed, because the other members of the family have no previous experience with facing this type of pressure from society. This difference leaves most LGBTQ individuals without effective advice or role models within the family structure, which could otherwise help them deal with this type of adversity. Furthermore, discrimination, in certain cases, can also come from their own family members, further compounding the negative impact it has on the individual.

Ideally, sexual identity would develop in an easily discussed and nurtured manner, much the same way that growth in academics, the arts, or sports is easily achieved in modern society. Most adolescents in the United States develop their sexual identity in a manner similar to that which their parents, teachers, mentors, and health care providers did: by trial and error without responsible and accurate sources of information readily available and openly provided. These maturing adolescents, seeking information and reassurance, discuss sexuality with their friends, watch the obligatory "health" movie(s), take in what they can get from the media, and possibly have the "birds-and-bees" talk with their parent(s). This is not to say that there is a pervasive, active attempt to avoid the provision of information regarding sexuality, but rather, the current culture does not allow easy or open discussion of these important issues. This process can be more complicated for the homosexual or questioning adolescent, because much of the information they access is geared to heterosexual youth, and questions about homosexuality may be considered taboo.[7]

VULNERABILITIES: PSYCHOLOGICAL AND PHYSICAL HEALTH RISKS

Research has demonstrated that high school students who self-identify as lesbian or bisexual are equally as likely as heterosexual women to have ever had vaginal intercourse; at the same time, they have a significantly higher rate of both pregnancy and a history of physical or sexual abuse.[8] Males with same-sex partners have an increased incidence of emotional distress and are less popular among heterosexual males, but they are popular with females. Both female and male bisexual youth have had the highest rate of risk factors identified.[9] Increased victimization, use of violence, drug use, and suicide attempts were seen in males with increasing numbers of male sexual partners, which is likely a result of the increased stress and peer disconnectedness.[10] Research has demonstrated an increased risk for suicidal ideation and suicide attempts in both males and females who had experienced same-sex relationships, whereas protective factors, including family connectedness, a sense that their school was safe, and the presence of another caring adult in their life, were effective in decreasing those odds.[11]

Suicidal ideation and behavior are extremely common among LGBTQ youth, with surveys indicating that ~42% have experienced suicidal ideation and 28% had made at least 1 or more suicide attempts during the preceding year.[12] Suicide is the leading cause of death among LGBTQ youth with estimates that they are at a two- to threefold increased risk of attempted suicide and may account for up to 30% of youth suicides annually. In addition to suicidal ideation and suicidality, risks such as early and frequent use of cocaine, early age of sexual initiation, marijuana use, tobacco use, increased number of sexual partners, having property stolen or damaged, and an overall increased risk of engagement in multiple risk behaviors is increased in LGBTQ youth when compared with the overall student population.

Understanding that protective factors decrease the likelihood of some of the types of harm described above ultimately makes much of the discomfort that providers feel in regards to these topics easier to understand. For an adolescent, having several trusted individuals in one's life provides the ability to discuss concerns and find collaborative solutions to the myriad problems encountered, which can be the first step in reducing the impact of stressful situations. These trusted individuals can be parents, teachers, mentors, peers, and health care providers. Although elements of society may remain biased against everyone who is not part of the majority viewpoint, causing increased stress to those in the minority, strength in numbers of supportive individuals can decrease that influence.

SEXUAL ATTRACTION: BEHAVIORS AND GENDER IDENTITY

To fully discuss this topic, a clear distinction needs to be drawn between gender identity and sexual identity. This critically important distinction has been confused historically, but they are not remotely connected and remain distinctly different issues. The following explanations are offered to help clarify some of the distinctions between the 2 issues.

Sexual Identity: Attraction and Behavior

An individual's personal assessment of his or her sexual orientation as heterosexual, homosexual, bisexual, or asexual is known as sexual identity. The development of these thoughts and desires causes stress to adolescents as they worry about how they view themselves and their position within society with respect to those issues and how to deal with sexual desire and activity. For clinicians, these thoughts can sometimes be unsettling and difficult to discuss, but it is clear that there is a need to find a way to discuss these issues for the sake of their patients. If the care provider is unable to do this without bias, the patient will need to be referred to someone who is able to treat those individuals without the possibility of overt or covert discrimination.

There can be discordance between sexual identity and sexual orientation and between self-identified sexual orientation and sexual behavior, which reveals that sexual identity does not predict sexual behavior.[13,14] The initial research regarding sexual orientation, based on studying sexual behavior, was conducted by Kinsey, who has remained a controversial figure from the time he began his work to the present day. His work revealed that in the period from puberty to age 20, 28% of boys and 17% of girls had 1 or more homosexual experiences. This work revealed that 37% of adults have had homosexual experiences and that 10% consider themselves predominantly homosexual in orientation.[15,16] This work, although widely quoted, praised, and criticized, started a public discussion with respect to sexual identity in the middle of the last century. A cross-sectional study conducted in adolescents revealed that of 13- to 19-year-olds, 11% of boys and 6% of girls reported at least 1 homosexual experience, with 17% of boys 16 to 19 years old reporting such activities.[17] This research revealed that 10.7% of high school students between 12 and 18 years of age were "unsure" of their sexual orientation. Approximately 5% to 6% of these students described same-sex attraction, and 1.1% of girls and 1.5% of boys described themselves as bisexual or homosexual.[18] This finding was further elucidated by using 3 characteristics to measure homosexuality and bisexuality: desire, identity, and behavior. A total of 2.4% of men and 1.3% of women defined their sexual orientation as homosexual or bisexual when they used all 3 categories as a guide. When defined by any 1 of these 3 components, 10.1% of men and 8.6% of women identified themselves as homosexual in orientation.[19]

Gender Identity

Gender refers to the behavioral, cultural, or psychological traits typically associated with 1 chromosomal (on the basis of genetic information) or phenotypic (on the basis of appearance) sex. For a parent or care provider, the phenotypic sex is typically discovered during the prenatal ultrasound or within seconds of a child's birth. Each individual begins to develop a perception of being male or female at approximately the second or third year of life, referred to as gender identity. In transgendered individuals, this sense of gender identity is incongruent with their chromosomal or phenotypic sex. The *Diagnostic and Statistical Manual of Mental Disorders, Fourth Edition* (DSM-IV TR) defines this incongruency as gender-identity dysphoria, which has 2 criteria: strong and persistent cross-gender identification and persistent discomfort about one's assigned gender or a sense of inappropriateness in the gender role of that sex. This is different from the commonly observed cross-gender behavior seen in children. According to parental reports, 6% of 4- to 5-year-old boys sometimes or frequently behaved like the opposite gender, although when the child was asked, only 1.3% wished to be female. For girls, 11.8% of 4- to 5-year-olds sometimes or frequently behaved like the opposite gender, whereas 5.0% wished to be male.[20] Without any intervention or therapy, the vast majority of both boys and girls who exhibit these types of behaviors grow to have their gender identity congruent with their chromosomal or phenotypic sex.

The prevalence of gender-identity disorder can be difficult to estimate. The DSM-IV-TR estimates that ~1 of 30 000 adult males and 1 of 100 000 adult females seek sex-reassignment surgery, which must be smaller than that of transgender individuals within society, because a relatively large number of individuals within the transgender community do not have genital surgery.[21] These numbers from the DSM have been questioned, and transsexual individuals may be more prevalent than 1 of 2500 males on the basis of those undergoing sex-reassignment surgery.[22] These numbers are likely underestimated because of a variety of factors including coexistent disorders, lifestyle choices, fluctuation in severity, and acceptance of gender-variant behavior.

SCREENING AND COUNSELING

Before embarking on a mission of evaluating any individual's sexual identity, sexual orientation, or gender identity, it is important to remember that the process of evaluation tends to lead to a formal labeling of the individual. In an ideal society, this type of label would be seen only as transient designation that will likely evolve or change with time. The word "adolescence" is derived from Latin, which literally means to grow up. It is a time of intense and constant change and is critically important and clinically relevant. An ill-timed or ill-chosen label, inadvertently given by a well-meaning care provider, can only add confusion to the future care of the patient. An overview of methods to help build the relationship and improve the clinic experience for everyone involved is detailed in Table 1.

Table 1
Important considerations for discussing sexual orientation and behaviors

Provide and ensure confidentiality
    Patient/provider time (without parent or guardian) at every visit
    Office/clinic policy statement for patients and parents to read
    Reason for visit may not be apparent until time alone is granted
Establish and maintain trust and respect
    Use gender- and orientation-neutral language
    Do not assume anyone's gender or sexual orientation
    Do not assume behaviors are a result of expressed orientation
    Allow discussions to progress from open-ended to specific questions
    Use appropriate follow-up questions to improve relationship
Demonstrate acceptance and openness
    Use appropriate displays, symbols, and materials throughout the office
    Provide pamphlets and/or literature in lobby and clinic rooms
    Discuss sensitivity with all patient-care staff

Confidentiality is the first and foremost consideration when it comes to the evaluation process. This type of trust is required for even the most superficial discussion of sexual identity and behavior to be remotely useful. For confidentiality to exist, it is necessary that a specific time during the patient encounter be provided, in which the clinical provider and adolescent can speak together without the parents or guardians. The right to confidentiality for adolescent health care visits has been supported by >20 different organizations that have a stake in the provision of top-quality health care for adolescents.[23]

There are no specific questions or methods to gather all the information that may be necessary to provide excellent care; rather, the discussion of sexuality and sexual behavior is best thought of as a process. For this process to be effective, it is important that both clinician and adolescent develop a trust and rapport with each other before sensitive questions are approached. Everyone develops her or her own style and approach to interacting with adolescents, although the information is still gained in a stepwise fashion. During the confidential time, selected usage of a semistructured interview can be helpful in initiating some of the discussions. A well-publicized approach that has been used successfully falls under the mnemonic HEEADSSSS (home, eating, education, alcohol, drugs and tobacco, suicidality and depression, safety, spirituality and sex).[24] This approach allows a transition from relatively easier subjects to more difficult subjects, with discussions concerning sexuality and sexual abuse at the very end of the list.

Caution must be exercised with an interaction style that relies on direct questions early in a discussion; this approach will often yield an "expected" answer rather than the factual answer. As with other personal issues, these very personal types of subjects can typically be approached by using indirect "trigger questions" such as "What are your thoughts about people your age having sex?" or "What kinds of activities do you include in having sex?" These types of questions will begin to elicit information about sexuality and sexual behavior. No question or set of questions can replace a series of conversations that provide the appropriate combination of honesty, depth, and usefulness to be of value. The only bad question is the one that is not asked. A recent survey of self-identified lesbian, gay, and bisexual youth revealed that although >70% of individuals were out (living openly with respect to their sexual orientation), <50% of them had ever been asked by their physician about their sexual orientation. The strongest response for how this should be accomplished was for the physician to "just ask."[25]

Another clinical caveat of which to be aware is the variability of the chief complaint listed for an office visit, when looking at clinic schedules, because some individuals will not describe the true nature of the visit to the person who schedules the appointment, either because of discomfort with discussing private matters with a relatively unknown stranger or for fear of reprisal from their parents or guardians. This is not an example of dishonesty but, rather, the mark of an astute individual who is forced to make decisions with very personal information. Discovering this information after the allotted clinic time has passed typically infuriates the care provider while, at the same time, delays or prevents the care the adolescent deserves. This type of situation can be avoided by asking early during the confidential portion of the visit if there is anything else that needs to be discussed outside the listed chief complaint. Working from the goal of the provision of the highest-quality care, it is easier to understand why someone might feel uncomfortable discussing personal matters when scheduling an appointment.

Trust is ultimately required for the management of any issues surrounding the area of sexual or gender identity, orientation, and behavior. Ongoing assurance and demonstration of confidentiality allows the best framework for trust to develop. Several factors can improve the perception of openness in the clinical arena, which have been well described.[26,27] Aligning the goals for each visit is important, and specific goals for each visit should be mutually agreed on by both the patient and care provider during the private portion of the visit.

It is important to remember that it is much less critical to diagnose anyone's gender or sexual orientation than it is to provide sound medical advice on the basis of current or impending risk behaviors. Altering the standard question from "Do you have sex with males, females, or both?" to "Can you tell me what you do with your sexual partner(s) or significant other(s)?" can provide entry into the discussion of sexual behavior and risk-factor assessment while minimizing any prejudices that may enter the conversation. In addition, it avoids the concept of labeling while focusing on the discussion of more immediate concerns. This approach allows the provision of confidential, factual, and nonjudgmental information in the context of awareness of the special considerations associated with caring for nonheterosexual and transgendered youth.[28]

For the clinician, although these discussions may be somewhat uncomfortable, it is important to remember that the adolescent who is discussing his or her thoughts, desires, or behaviors may have never discussed them with anyone in a position of authority. It is important to reiterate that these types of feelings may be transient or lifelong and may or may not reflect adult sexual orientation. A supportive and helpful approach will ultimately serve those who have placed their trust with their provider, to think through and discuss these feelings and any current or potential future actions. One common experience typically occurs when the individual feels some permanence with respect to these types of feelings and considers informing his or her family and friends who have not yet been told of the individual's sexual orientation. This process, typically referred to as "coming out," can be empowering to the individual if it goes well, but it can also be devastating or dangerous depending on the reaction of those who hear this information. A physician's involvement in the process can be extremely useful to the patient. It also cannot be overstated that providing support for parents during this time of stress can be immensely important.

Table 2
Selected sources for additional information

American Academy of Pediatrics (www.aap.org)
  Gay, Lesbian, and Bisexual Teens: Facts for Teens and Their Parents Brochure (available from the American Academy of Pediatrics bookstore; www.aap.org/bookstore)
Centers for Disease Control and Prevention: lesbian, gay, bisexual, and transgender health (www.cdc.gov/lgbthealth)
Gay and Lesbian Medical Association (www.glma.org)
McMaster University: wellness health care information resources (http://hsl.mcmaster.ca/tomflem/gay.html)
Parents, Families, and Friends of Lesbians and Gays (www.pflag.org)

Successful navigation through the transitions of adolescence leads to a more rewarding and successful life as an adult. Unresolved issues and insecurities undermine successful transition to adulthood and carry with them a great deal of emotional baggage. Issues that surround sexual identity and behavior can yield increased rates of delinquency, suicidality, substance abuse, sexually transmitted diseases, and undesired pregnancy. Isolation or fear of isolation from friends and/or family secondary to real or even perceived discrimination and/or disappointment makes sexual identity formation all the more difficult.

Several sources of information can provide additional guidance to both adolescent patients and their families (see Table 2 for sources of information). Having handouts or informational pamphlets from these various sources in the office setting demonstrates not only sensitivity in this area but also provides information that can be further explored outside the office visit.

As a care provider, it is imperative that personal judgments or biases should never be imposed on an individual patient. It is important to provide thoughtful and accurate information from which maturing adolescents can make their own decision regarding the life they will lead. This provision of sound and competent advice is the goal of every provider. A patient who is able to follow the advice will most likely see a benefit in both health and well-being. If adolescents are not able to adhere to the advice initially, the provision of follow-up appointments will help further establish and promote trust in the health care relationship and will likely provide a benefit to them in the end.

REFERENCES

1. Friedman RC, Downey JI. Homosexuality. N Engl J Med. 1994;331:923–930
2. Livingood JM, ed. National Institute of Mental Health, Task Force on Homosexuality Final Report and Background Papers. Rockville, MD: Department of Health, Education and Welfare; 1976. Publication 76-357
3. Levay S. A difference in hypothalamic structure between heterosexual and homosexual men. Science. 1991;253:1034–1037

4. Blackless M, Charuvastra A, Derryck A, Fausto-Sterling A, Lauzanne K, Lee E. How sexually dimorphic are we? Review and synthesis. *Am J Hum Biol.* 2000;12:151–166
5. Savic I, Berglund H, Lindström P. Brain response to putative phermones in homosexual men. *Proc Natl Acad Sci U S A.* 2005;102:7356–7361
6. Carrion VG, Lock J. The coming out process: developmental stages for sexual minority youth. *Clin Child Psychol Psychiatry.* 1997;2:369–377
7. Floyd FJ, Stein TS. Sexual orientation identity formation among gay, lesbian, and bisexual youths: multiple patterns of milestone experiences. *J Res Adolesc.* 2002;12:167–191
8. Saewyc EM, Bearinger LH, Blum RW, Resnick MD. Sexual intercourse, abuse, and pregnancy among adolescent women: does sexual orientation make a difference? *Fam Plann Perspect.* 1999;31:127–131
9. Udry JR, Chantala K. Risk assessment of adolescents with same-sex relationships. *J Adolesc Health.* 2002;31:84–92
10. DuRant RH, Krowchuk DP, Sinal SH. Victimization, use of violence, and drug use at school among male adolescents who engage in same-sex sexual behavior. *J Pediatr.* 1998;133:113–118
11. Eisenberg ME, Resnick MD. Suicidality among gay, lesbian and bisexual youth: the role of protective factors. *J Adolesc Health.* 2006;39:662–668
12. Garofalo R, Wolf RC, Kessel S, Palfrey SJ, DuRant RH. The association between health risk behaviors and sexual orientation among a school-based sample of adolescents. *Pediatrics.* 1998;101:895–902
13. Ross MW, Essien EJ, Williams ML, Fernandez-Esquer ME. Concordance between sexual behavior and sexual identity in street outreach samples of four racial/ethnic groups. *Sex Transm Dis.* 2003;30:110–113
14. Pathela P, Hajat A, Schillinger J, Blank S, Sell R, Mostashari F. Discordance between sexual behavior and self-reported sexual identity: a population-based survey of New York City men. *Ann Intern Med.* 2006;145:416–425
15. Institute for Sex Research. *Sexual Behavior in the Human Male.* Kinsey AC, Pomeroy WB, Martin CE, eds. Philadelphia, PA: WB Saunders; 1948
16. Institute for Sex Research. *Sexual Behavior in the Human Female.* Kinsey AC, Pomeroy WB, Martin CE, Gebhard PH, eds. Philadelphia, PA: WB Saunders; 1953
17. Sorensen RC. *Adolescent Sexuality in Contemporary America.* New York, NY: World Publishing; 1973
18. Remafedi G, Resnick M, Blum R, Harris L. Demography of sexual orientation in adolescents. *Pediatrics.* 1992;89:714–721
19. Laumann EO, Gagnon JH, Michael RT, Michaels S. *The Social Organization of Sexuality: Sexual Practices in the United States.* Chicago, IL: University of Chicago Press; 1994
20. Bradley SJ, Zucker KJ. Gender identity disorder: a review of the past 10 years [published correction appears in *J Am Acad Child Adolesc Psychiatry.* 1997;36:1310.] *J Am Acad Child Adolesc Psychiatry.* 1997;36:872–880
21. American Psychiatric Association. *DSM-IV-TR, Diagnostic and Statistical Manual of Mental Disorders,* 4th ed. Text revision. Washington, DC: American Psychiatric Association; 2000
22. Conway L. How frequently does transsexualism occur? Available at: http://ai.eecs.umich.edu/people/conway/TS/TSprevalence.html. Accessed July 20, 2007
23. Morreale, MC, Stinnett AJ, and Dowling, EC, eds. *Policy Compendium on Confidential Health Services for Adolescents,* 2nd ed. Chapel Hill, NC: Center for Adolescent Health and the Law; 2005
24. Goldenring J, Rosen D. Getting into adolescent heads: an essential update. *Contemp Pediatr.* 2004;21:64–90
25. Meckler GD, Elliott MN, Kanouse DE, Beals KP, Schuster MA. Nondisclosure of sexual orientation to a physician among a sample of gay, lesbian, and bisexual youth. *Arch Pediatr Adolesc Med.* 2006;160:1248–1254
26. Catallozzi M, Rudy BJ. Lesbian, gay, bisexual, transgendered, and questioning youth: the importance of a sensitive and confidential sexual history in identifying the risk and implementing treatment for sexually transmitted infections. *Adolesc Med Clin.* 2004;15:353–367

27. Gay and Lesbian Medical Association. Guidelines for care of lesbian, gay, bisexual, and transgendered patients. Available at: http://ce54.citysoft.com/_data/n_0001/resources/live/GLMA%20guidelines%202006%20FINAL.pdf. Accessed July 20, 2007
28. Frankowski BL; American Academy of Pediatrics, Committee on Adolescence. *Pediatrics*. 2004;113:1827–1832

Sexual Health of Adolescents With Chronic Health Conditions

Lynn Rew, EdD, RN, AHN-BC, FAAN

Department of Nursing, University of Texas, 1700 Red River, Austin, TX 78701, USA

Sexual health reflects a synthesis of genetic determination, physiologic function, gender identity, social roles, and behaviors related to sexuality. During adolescence, sexual health is a major focus as the individual becomes a physically mature person who is capable of sexual reproduction and becomes cognitively and socially aware of gender roles and responsibilities for behaviors.[1] For all adolescents, risk behaviors can jeopardize health either directly or indirectly and increase the potential for morbidity and even mortality.[2] Health risk behaviors are known to increase with age, vary by gender, and occur in clusters.[3–5] Whereas risk-taking is considered part of normal adolescent development, it is of special concern for adolescents who have chronic health conditions (CHCs), because they may have greater potential for adverse health outcomes than their able-bodied peers.[6] Because of improved treatment and care for life-threatening pediatric conditions and illnesses, the prevalence of CHCs in children and young adults has increased in the last 3 decades.[7] Other influences of equal importance include genetic susceptibility and social environmental factors.[8] Thus, the percentage of teenagers with CHCs presenting to primary care practices will continue to become more common. Thus, it is important for primary care providers to understand what is known about health risk behaviors in adolescents with CHCs, identify aspects of these conditions that affect sexual health, and be familiar with the recommendations about anticipatory sexual guidance for this special group of adolescents.

HEALTH RISK BEHAVIORS IN ADOLESCENTS WITH CHCS

Few researchers have addressed the relationship between having a CHC and engaging in risk behaviors during adolescence, particularly behaviors that directly affect sexual health. Analyzing data from a representative sample of 20 780 American adolescents in the National Longitudinal Study of Adolescent Health, researchers found that youth with disabilities were significantly more

---

*Corresponding author.
E-mail address*: ellerew@mail.utexas.edu (L. Rew)

involved in health risk behaviors, including early sexual intercourse, than their peers.[9] More specifically, those youth with emotional disabilities (eg, feeling blue, depressed, fearful, or lonely) were significantly more likely than those without to engage in regular alcohol and marijuana use, smoking and suicide attempts and to report first sexual intercourse before 12 years of age.

National data that compared adolescents with asthma and those without have shown that youth with asthma used substances (eg, cigarettes, marijuana, inhalants) at rates that were equal to or greater than those without this condition.[10] Similarly, adolescent survivors of childhood cancer reported health risk behaviors of lifetime cigarette use, lack of physical activity, and insufficient sun protection that were similar to those of healthy peers.[11]

Already sensing their vulnerability, some teenagers with CHCs may engage in fewer risk behaviors as a result of less unsupervised time.[12] One sample of teenagers with chronic illnesses, when compared with those without, showed less antisocial behavior and less substance use, but they were also less psychosexually and socially developed than normal peers. On one hand, parents might be more involved with these youth, thus giving them less unsupervised time. On the other hand, some reports have suggested that adolescents with CHCs may exhibit more risk behaviors to compensate for all the restrictions imposed.[13]

In their review of peer influences on youth with CHCs, researchers found that peer relationships may affect health risk behaviors both negatively and positively.[14] In particular, peers influenced the initiation and continuation of smoking and cessation in teenagers with CHCs. Although reports of alcohol use were fewer than their peers, teenagers with CHCs had rates of alcohol use that were still relatively high, a behavior particularly deleterious to youth with, for example, cystic fibrosis (CF) or diabetes mellitus (DM). This review also showed that those who had a low rate of social support engaged in more risky sexual behaviors and had more sexually transmitted infections (STIs) than their peers. On a more positive note, adolescents with DM who exhibited poor metabolic control reported that peers also helped them to exercise regularly.

In summary, the literature on whether health risk behaviors, including sexual behaviors, are increased or decreased in adolescents with CHCs is equivocal. There is some evidence, however, that additional protective factors such as social support and peer influence may mitigate circumstances with increased risk.

INFLUENCES OF CHCS ON PHYSICAL AND PSYCHOSOCIAL DEVELOPMENT

Chronic disorders affect ~2 million adolescents in this country and account for a variety of physical, mental, and social disabilities. CHCs can have biological, cognitive, or psychological characteristics, and they can last or are expected to last a minimum of 12 months. Consequences of having CHCs can result in relative functional limitations, with the adolescent having to rely on assistance in the form of medications or assistive devices.[15] A more common criterion used in a national study is whether the child or adolescent has a condition that limits usual daily activities. This criterion currently identifies ~7% of children and adolescents as having this condition.[8] Factors that have an effect on the impact of a CHC on the development of the adolescent include (1) age at onset of the condition, (2) duration and visibility of the condition, (3) comorbid conditions, (4) expected course of the disorder, (5) and expected rate of survival. These factors may impose developmental limitations on the individual that can affect physical, cognitive, emotional, and social development and functioning.[15]

PHYSICAL DEVELOPMENT AND FUNCTIONING

As indicated by Biro et al[16], defining pubertal maturation includes the stage (sequence), age at onset (timing), and rate of progression (tempo). There are conditions that occur during adolescence that are primarily behaviorally induced but still may be chronic. Conditions such as disordered eating and substance use disorders have the potential to affect puberty and reproductive function, depending on the age of onset of the condition and the stage of development of puberty.[4,17,18]

Some CHCs affect pubertal timing more than others. For example, adolescents with spina bifida often experience early or precocious puberty.[19] A multicenter study of 207 children and adolescents with cerebral palsy with moderate-to-severe motor impairment found, specifically for white children, that puberty began earlier compared with the general population, but menarche often occurred later.[20] Similarly, girls with CF also had delayed menarche with a median age of 13.9 years compared with the average age of the population of 12.8 years old.[21] In males with CF, irregular development of the reproductive tract often leads to infertility.[22] Adolescents with type 1 diabetes have also been shown to have impaired physical growth and delayed sexual maturation, which is probably related to less-than-optimal glycemic control in childhood.[23]

Both males and females with epilepsy have been found to have impaired sexual development. For example, in Egypt, 130 males with epilepsy were compared with 63 healthy males. Those with epilepsy were found to be significantly shorter and to have significantly reduced penile length and testicular volume.[24] These findings were independent of the length of duration of the condition. Similarly, 66 females with epilepsy from the same clinic were compared with 40 control adolescents. Those with diagnosed epilepsy were found to be shorter and to have a higher incidence of obesity than the girls in the control group. Those girls who were already postmenarchal had a high prevalence of polycystic ovarian syndrome.[25] In addition to affecting the timing of puberty, CHCs may affect sexual functioning in adolescence and early adulthood. For example, males with spina bifida have reported erectile and urinary problems that inhibited their sexual activity.[26]

Overall, this limited evidence suggests that many adolescents with CHCs experience variations in age at onset (timing) and even the rate of progression (tempo) of pubertal development. This variation places them out of synchrony with their peers, which can potentially lead to difficulties in social relationships and increase the likelihood that they will engage in sexual and other health-harming behaviors.

COGNITIVE FUNCTIONING

Adolescents with CHCs may experience impaired cognitive abilities related to the pathophysiology of their condition, its treatment, or lack of appropriate management. Issues of care and treatment may result in not only missed time in school but barriers to obtaining the necessary resources to learn in the school setting. In a review of literature concerning CHCs and student performance at school, patients with diabetes, epilepsy, and sickle cell anemia, in particular, had at least some decline in cognitive ability and academic achievement, which was probably related to a combination of issues involving the disease, lack of good control, and/or complications from medications required for treatment.[27] Patients with neurofibromatosis type 1 are frequently also diagnosed with learning disabilities.[28] Youth with juvenile primary fibromyalgia syndrome may experience cognitive dysfunction associated with chronic pain and fatigue.[29] Adolescents who have survived childhood cancer may have decreased levels of general intelligence and academic achievement, particularly if treatment involved radiation or chemotherapy to the central nervous system and some delays related to missing school.[30,31] In 1 recently published long-term follow-up study of >1300 childhood cancer survivors, 75% of them had at least 1 or more adverse health outcomes from the list of psychosocial/cognitive problems the group most commonly mentioned in their research.[32] Recent guidelines and recommendations for screening and managing these neurocognitive problems have been published.[33] Similarly, children diagnosed with asthma reportedly miss school twice as often as children who do not have it.[34] In a national study of teenagers living in Canada, a subsample of 213 adolescents with arthritis or rheumatism reported a lower enrollment in school compared with those without these conditions.[35] Thus, missing school and/or being in school without the appropriate support often translates into loss of both formal (ie, classroom) and informal (ie, peer-led) experiences, which can affect sexuality education.

Self-management for some chronic conditions such as diabetes and epilepsy is more complex and requires cognitive capabilities that are fully intact. Such self-care requires not only education and knowledge but also the ability to apply the information to minimize complications. For all teenagers with CHCs, preventing unplanned pregnancies and STIs becomes even more important, because a pregnancy has the potential to exacerbate CHCs, as does an unsuspected, thus undiagnosed, sexually acquired infection. A study of 80 female adolescents with DM and 37 matched healthy controls found that those with DM reported their first sexual intercourse at a mean age of 15.7 years compared with those without DM at a mean age of 16.1 years. The study also indicated that teenagers lacked important information that would help them prevent unplanned pregnancy and its complications.[36] Similarly, researchers conducted a national survey of 459 patients from 20 hemophilia treatment centers and 8 hemophilia associations. Nearly 25% of the 110 respondents were between the ages of 13 and 21 years. Although hepatitis and HIV were among the top 4 concerns of this group, 78% did not know all of the ways in which hepatitis B and C could be transmitted. These researchers concluded that these youth needed to understand more about the risks related to sexual activity, and they encouraged greater efforts toward educating them about varied disease transmission routes.[37]

SOCIAL/DEVELOPMENT AND EMOTIONAL FUNCTIONING

Social relationships in adolescence are critical for optimal development. Adolescents with some CHCs are excluded from the usual teenaged culture because of the stigma associated with their condition.[38] Others may be excluded because of the limitations imposed by characteristic problems such as chronic pain, disrupted sleep, and increased irritability related to their primary illness.[29]

From a literature review of adolescents with cerebral palsy who also had normal levels of intelligence, Wiegerink et al[39] concluded that youth with cerebral palsy had less exposure to peer culture, less active social lives, and delayed dating when compared with their peers. They also found that these youth had fewer sexual relationships than their able-bodied peers, which was related to lower self-efficacy and sexual self-esteem. Similarly, teenagers with juvenile fibromyalgia syndrome reported being less popular than their healthy peers and had few reciprocated friendships.[40]

Mood swings related to pubertal development are experienced to some extent by many adolescents, including those with and without a CHC. Having a mood disorder such as depression or bipolar disease that is particularly undiagnosed or inadequately treated often leads to exacerbation of these mood swings. Controlling for demographics, Asarnow et al[41] found that adolescents with depression were more likely to have another chronic condition such as asthma, arthritis, chronic bronchitis, epilepsy, and/or diabetes. Parents of adolescents with diabetes, for example, expressed concern that having diabetes added burdens to their children's lives and interrupted family dynamics.[42] Similarly, researchers have noted that having a chronic disease throughout childhood can interfere with the successful completion of developmental tasks during adolescence and lower one's quality of life.[13] Adolescents with juvenile idiopathic arthritis (JIA) have also expressed concern about the burden that their condition can place on caregivers. The longer the duration of this condition, the more likely these children were to experience a psychiatric condition such as depressive disorder, somatoform disorder, adjustment disorder, or mixed anxiety and depressive disorder.[43] Adolescents with JIA also experience psychosocial problems related to negative body image, have often reported that they feel different than their peers, and have concerns about discrimination.[44] These reports are similar to those of other adolescents with CHCs who have symptoms of increased risk of anxiety and depression and feel different than their peers.[28]

SUMMARY OF INFLUENCES

Many adolescents with CHCs experience challenges in physical, cognitive, emotional, and social functioning. Some CHCs affect children's pubertal timing and tempo, with earlier or later onset of puberty than their healthy peers and implications for social and emotional functioning. Others have reduced neurocognitive function related to disease or conditions, the treatment they receive, and/or poor control. Poor school attendance and impaired socialization result in poor school performance and academic development that further isolate teenagers from activities and healthy relationships. Adolescents with limited mobility and decreased opportunities to interact with peers may seek socialization experiences through the use of Internet Web sites.[45] The article by English[46] in this issue of *AM:STARs* reflects on the reported exposures to the media that adolescents report (both desired and unwanted) to sexually oriented or sexually explicit Web sites that may impact their sexual socialization. Involvement with the Internet may become the teenager's major source of information and interaction. How the Internet impacts or relates to health risk behaviors in teenagers with CHCs is not currently known, nor has it been adequately studied.

GUIDANCE AND COUNSELING FOR SEXUAL HEALTH

Researchers have shown that many healthy adolescent girls do not share with primary care providers that they are sexually active. Thus, screening for STIs, performing pelvic examinations when indicated, and counseling about safe sex and pregnancy prevention do not occur.[47] Yet, guidelines for providing preventive health care for the adolescent age group include asking about substance use, depressive symptoms, and sexual activity.[48] Counseling youth about the prevention of pregnancy and STIs should begin before their sexual debut, which for many may be before they are 14 years old.[49] Urine-based screening for common STIs such as chlamydia and gonorrhea is recommended for sexually experienced adolescents, including those who have CHCs and report that they are sexually active.[50] Asking teenagers about sources of information such as their favorite Web sites may offer some clues about the quality and quantity of information they receive.

Before providers can ask questions that involve sexual health, they need to assess their own attitudes and knowledge. Special training of designated professionals in this area may help to ensure that information offered by the health care provider is both correct and appropriate for the teenager and his or her family.[51] Previous surveys have indicated that adolescents with CHCs acknowledge that medical specialists knew a lot about their disease conditions, but they rarely discussed other issues or concerns such as sexual health.[52] For example, having a parent or another health professional remain in the examining room at all times with an adolescent is viewed as a significant barrier to the discussion of sensitive topics, which might include fertility concerns, contraception, and STI prevention and detection.[18,53]

In studies of urban teenagers, the majority of participants (73%) reported talking with a health care provider about at least 1 sexual health topic, but this portion still remains below the recommended guidelines.[54] In another study of teenagers from low-income families in New York, a survey that used a random-digit dialing system determined that the reported prevalence of counseling about health risk behaviors was low (eg, 17% were counseled about depression, and 32% were asked about alcohol use), and just over half (52%) were queried about the risk for STIs. More girls than boys in this study reported receiving counseling for birth control.[55] Neither of these studies included data concerning the health status of participants.

In a study of sexual and reproductive health of young adult men with CF, Sawyer et al[22] asked the participants when they first discussed fertility. The data provided by the participants indicated that the age at which their first discussion of fertility took place ranged from age 7 to age 31 years, with a mean age of 16.4 years. Those surveyed suggested that age 14.4 years would have been more appropriate. Those who were older when they were first told about possible infertility reported being more upset than those who were told at an earlier age. These researchers also found that when the participants were adolescents, 30% of their sample thought they did not need to use a condom, and they often confused infertility with impotence. Twenty-two percent of the men in this sample reported that infertility had affected some of their personal relationships. The researchers underscored the importance of health professionals in initiating the discussion about fertility with young males who have CF and should include a semen analysis. As another example, a review of studies was published that addressed the effectiveness of psychoeducational interventions with children and adolescents who had asthma, cancer, chronic fatigue syndrome, diabetes, or JIA. Most of the interventions and education addressed disease management, family functioning, knowledge, psychosocial well-being, self-efficacy, pain, and metabolic control. There were no interventions or educational approaches offered for sexuality issues.[56]

CONCLUSIONS

Adolescents with CHCs share a common stage of development with adolescents without such conditions, yet many of these conditions affect their physical and sexual maturation and cognitive, emotional, and social functioning. Much of what is known about these variations as they relate to CHCs is based on small samples and from studies performed in countries other than the United States. There is clear evidence that adolescents with CHCs engage in the same health risk behaviors as their healthy peers. Although health care professionals and parents must pay close attention to the particular aspects of managing CHCs in adolescents, there is mounting evidence that these youngsters have physical, cognitive, and psychosocial needs related to becoming sexually mature and responsible individuals that also warrant close attention. Sexuality education must be provided and modified by parents and professionals at every opportunity. Peer relationships may also help or hinder the development of healthy behaviors of youth, and health care providers must remain alert for indicators of dysfunction. In addition, it is important to continue to encourage developmentally appropriate family support, particularly because adolescents with CHCs who have good relationships within their families are likely to improve the chances of good health and psychosexual outcomes.[9]

The relationship between CHCs and various aspects of development affects the guidance and counseling provided to parents and health care providers. Health care providers hold unique social roles that require them to offer guidance and support for adolescents as they navigate the issues related to the development of sexual health amid the concerns and dilemmas of their CHCs. Sexuality information should be developmentally appropriate and be combined with the positive support of family, peers, and their environment. Support in making informed choices will help protect these teenagers from making choices that may lead to the development of other disabilities that might relate to the negative consequences of health risk behaviors.

REFERENCES

1. Rew L. Sexual health promotion in adolescents with chronic health conditions. *Fam Community Health*. 2006;29 (suppl 1):61S–69S
2. Rew L. *Adolescent Health: A Multidisciplinary Approach to Theory, Research, and Intervention*. Thousand Oaks, CA: Sage; 2005
3. Andrews JA, Tildesley E, Hops H, Duncan SC, Severson HH. Elementary school age children's future intentions and use of substances. *J Clin Child Adolesc Psychol*. 2003;32:556–567
4. Halpern CT, Kaestle CE, Hallfors DD. Perceived physical maturity, age of romantic partner, and adolescent risk behavior. *Prev Sci*. 2007;8:1–10
5. Maes L, Lievens J. Can the school make a difference? A multilevel analysis of adolescent risk and health behaviour. *Soc Sci Med*. 2003;56:517–529
6. Sawyer SM, Drew S, Yeo MS, Britto MT. Adolescents with a chronic condition: challenges living, challenges treating. *Lancet*. 2007;369:1481–1489
7. Van der lee JH, Mokkink LB, Grootenhuis MA, Heymans HS, Offringa M. Definitions and measurement of chronic health conditions of childhood. *JAMA*. 2007;297:2741–2751

8. Perrin JM, Bloom SR, Gortmaker SL. The increase of childhood chronic conditions in the United States. *JAMA.* 2007;297:2755–2759
9. Blum RW, Kelly A, Ireland M. Health-risk behaviors and protective factors among adolescents with mobility impairments and learning and emotional disabilities. *J Adolesc Health.* 2001;28: 481–490
10. Jones SE, Merkle S, Wheeler L, Mannino DM, Crossett L. Tobacco and other drug use among high school students with asthma. *J Adolesc Health.* 2006;39:291–294
11. Tercyak KP, Donze JR, Prahlad S, Mosher RB, Shad AT. Multiple behavioral risk factors among adolescent survivors of childhood cancer in the Survivor Health and Resilience Education (SHARE) program. *Pediatr Blood Cancer.* 2006;47:825–830
12. Stam H, Hartman EE, Deurloo JA, Groothoff J, Grootenhuis MA. Young adult patients with a history of pediatric disease: impact on course of life and transition into adulthood. *J Adolesc Health.* 2006;39:4–13
13. Grootenhuis MA, Stam H, Last BF, Groothoff JW. The impact of delayed development on the quality of life of adults with end-stage renal disease since childhood. *Pediatr Nephrol.* 2006;21: 538–544
14. La Greca AM, Bearman KJ, Moore H. Peer relations of youth with pediatric conditions and health risks: promoting social support and healthy lifestyles. *J Dev Behav Pediatr.* 2002;23:271–280
15. Coupey SM, Neinstein LS, Zeltzer LK. Chronic illness in the adolescent. In: Neinstein LS, ed. *Adolescent Health Care: A Practical Guide.* 4th ed. Philadelphia, PA: Lippincott, Williams & Wilkins; 2002:1511–1536
16. Biro FM. Puberty. *Adolesc Med.* 2007;18:425–433
17. McCabe MP, Ricciardelli LA. A longitudinal study of pubertal timing and extreme body change behaviors among adolescent boys and girls. *Adolescence.* 2004;39:145–166
18. Manlove JS, Ryan S, Franzetta K. Risk and protective factors associated with the transition to a first sexual relationship with an older partner. *J Adolesc Health.* 2007;40:135–143
19. Coakley RM, Holmbeck GN, Friedman D, Greenley RN, Thill AW. A longitudinal study of pubertal timing, parent-child conflict, and cohesion in families of young adolescents with spina bifida. *J Pediatr Psychol.* 2002;27:461–473
20. Worley G, Houlihan CM, Herman-Giddens ME, et al. Secondary sexual characteristics in children with cerebral palsy and moderate to severe motor impairment: a cross-sectional survey. *Pediatrics.* 2002;110:897–902
21. Stallings VA, Tomezsko, JL, Schall JI, et al. Adolescent development and energy expenditure in females with cystic fibrosis. *Clin Nutr.* 2005;24:737–745
22. Sawyer SM, Farrant B, Cerritelli B, Wilson J. A survey of sexual and reproductive health in men with cystic fibrosis: new challenges for adolescent and adult services. *Thorax.* 2005;60:326–330
23. Elamin A, Hussein O, Tuvemo T. Growth, puberty, and final height in children with type 1 diabetes. *J Diabetes Complicat.* 2006;20:252–256
24. El-Khayat HA, Shatla HM, Ali GK, Abdulgani MO, Tomoum HY, Attya HA. Physical and hormonal profile of male sexual development in epilepsy. *Epilepsia.* 2003;44:447–452
25. El-Khayat HA, Abd El-Basset FZ, Tomoum HY, et al. Physical growth and endocrine disorders during pubertal maturation in girls with epilepsy. *Epilepsia.* 2004;45:1106–1115
26. Nehring WM, Faux SA. Transitional and health issues of adults with neural tube defects. *J Nurs Scholarsh.* 2006;38;63–70
27. Taras H, Potts-Datema W. Chronic health conditions and student performance at school. *J Sch Health.* 2005;75:255–266
28. Sebold CD, Lovell A, Hopkin R, Noll R, Schorry E. Perception of disease severity in adolescents diagnosed with neurofibromatosis type 1. *J Adolesc Health.* 2004;35:297–302
29. Varni JW, Burwinkle TM, Limbers CA, Szer IS. The PedsQL as a patient-reported outcome in children and adolescents with fibromyalgia: an analysis of OMERACT domains. *Health Qual Life Outcomes.* 2007;5:9. Available at: www.hqlo.com/content/5/1/9. Accessed May 1, 2007
30. Moore IM. Cancer in children. In: Hayman LL, Mahon MM, Turner JR, eds. *Chronic Illness in Children: An Evidence-Based Approach.* New York, NY: Springer; 2002:80–103

31. Evan EE, Kaufman M, Cook AB, Zeltzer LK. Sexual health and self-esteem in adolescents and young adults with cancer. *Cancer.* 2006;107(suppl 7):1672–1679
32. Geenen MM, Cardous-Ubbink MC, Kremer LC, et al. Medical assessment of adverse health outcomes in long-term survivors of childhood cancer. *JAMA.* 2007;297:2705–2715
33. Nathan PC, Patel SK, Dilley K, et al. Guidelines for identification of, advocacy for, and intervention in neurocognitive problems in survivors of childhood cancer. *Arch Pediatr Adolesc Med.* 2007;161:798–806
34. Turner-Henson A, Johnston J. Pediatric asthma. In: Hayman LL, Mahon MM, Turner JR, eds. *Chronic Illness in Children: An Evidence-Based Approach.* New York, NY: Springer; 2002:3–26
35. Adam V, St-Pierre Y, Fautrel B, Clarke AE, Duffy CM, Penrod JR. What is the impact of adolescent arthritis and rheumatism? Evidence from a national sample of Canadians. *J Rheumatol.* 2005;32:354–361
36. Charron-Prochownik D, Sereika SM, Falsetti D, et al. Knowledge, attitudes, and behaviors related to sexuality and family planning in adolescent women with and without diabetes. *Pediatr Diabetes.* 2006;7:267–273
37. Nazzaro AM, Owens S, Hoots WK, Larson KL. Knowledge, attitudes, and behaviors of youths in the US hemophilia population: results of a national survey. *Am J Public Health.* 2006;96: 1618–1622
38. Cheung C, Wirrell E. Adolescents' perception of epilepsy compared with other chronic diseases: "through a teenager's eyes." *J Child Neurol.* 2006;21:214–222
39. Wiegerink DJ, Roebroeck ME, Donkervoort M, Stam HJ, Cohen-Kettenis PT. Social and sexual relationships of adolescents and young adults with cerebral palsy: a review. *Clin Rehabil.* 2006;20:1023–1031
40. Kashikar-Zuck S, Lynch AM, Graham TB, Swain NF, Mullen SM, Noll RB. Social functioning and peer relationships of adolescents with juvenile fibromyalgia syndrome. *Arthritis Rheum.* 2007;57:474–480
41. Asarnow JR, Jaycox LH, Duan N, et al. Depression and role impairment among adolescents in primary care clinics. *J Adolesc Health.* 2005;37:477–483
42. Carroll AE, Marrero DG. How do parents perceive their adolescent's diabetes: a qualitative study. *Diabet Med.* 2006;23:1222–1224
43. Mullick MS, Nahar, JS, Haq SA. Psychiatric morbidity, stressors, impact, and burden in juvenile idiopathic arthritis. *J Health Popul Nutr.* 2005;23:142–149
44. Shaw KL, Southwood TR, McDonagh JE; British Paediatric Rheumatology Group. User perspectives of transitional care for adolescents with juvenile idiopathic arthritis. *Rheumatology (Oxford).* 2004;43:770–778
45. Cameron KA, Salazar LF, Bernhardt JM, Burgess-Whitman N, Wingood GM, DiClemente RJ. Adolescents' experience with sex on the Web: results from online focus groups. *J Adolesc.* 2005;28:535–540
46. English A. Sexual and reproductive health care for adolescents: legal rights and policy challenges. *Adolesc Med.* 2007;18:571–581
47. McKee MD, Fletcher J, Schechter CB. Predictors of timely initiation of gynecologic care among urban adolescent girls. *J Adolesc Health.* 2006;39:183–191
48. Elster AB, Kuznets NJ. AMA Guidelines for Adolescent Preventive Services (GAPS): Recommendations and Rationale. Baltimore, MD: Williams & Wilkins; 1994
49. Rand CM, Auinger P, Klein JD, Weitzman M. Preventive counseling at adolescent ambulatory visits. *J Adolesc Health.* 2005;37:87–93
50. Asbel LE, Newbern C, Salmon M, Spain CV, Goldberg M. School-based screening for *Chlamydia trachomatis* and *Neisseria gonorrhoeae* among Philadelphia public high school students. *Sex Transm Dis.* 2006;33:614–620
51. Suris JC, Michaud PA, Viner R. The adolescent with a chronic condition, part I: developmental issues. *Arch Dis Child.* 2004;89:938–942
52. Kyngäs H. Patient education: perspective of adolescents with a chronic disease. *J Clin Nurs.* 2003;12:744–751

53. Beresford BA, Sloper P. Chronically ill adolescents' experiences of communicating with doctors: a qualitative study. *J Adolesc Health.* 2003;33:172–179
54. Merzel CR, Vandevanter NL, Middlestadt S, Bleakley A, Ledsky R, Messeri PA. Attitudinal and contextual factors associated with discussion of sexual issues during adolescent health visits. *J Adolesc Health.* 2004;35:108–115
55. Fairbrother G, Scheinmann R, Osthimer B, et al. Factors that influence adolescent reports of counseling by physicians on risky behavior. *J Adolesc Health.* 2005;37:467–476
56. Barlow JH, Ellard DR. Psycho-educational interventions for children with chronic disease, parents and siblings: an overview of the research evidence base. *Child Care Health Dev.* 2004;30:637–645

Relationship Violence in Adolescence

Alison J. Lin, MPH[a], Marissa Raymond, MPH[a],
Marina Catallozzi, MD[a,b], Owen Ryan, MPH, MIA[a],
Vaughn I. Rickert, PsyD[a,b]

[a]*Heilbrunn Department of Population and Family Health, Mailman School of Public Health, Columbia University, 60 Haven Ave B-2, New York, NY 10032, USA*

[b]*Department of Pediatrics, College of Physicians and Surgeons, Columbia University, 4th Floor, Room 449, New York, NY 10032, USA*

Adolescents' experiences with intimacy rapidly expand as they mature from children to young adults. While friendships deepen and romantic relationships form, some youth experience sexual harassment and coercion from peers as well as violence from dating and/or sexual partners. As discussed in "Development of Intimate Relationships in Adolescence"[1] later in this issue, relationships with peers, family, and romantic partners build on one another as adolescents develop the skills to engage in romantic relationships. Although this progression seems straightforward, many factors contribute to the relative success of adolescents' relationships that may affect their health.

Relationship violence among adolescents includes bullying, sexual harassment, dating violence, and/or coercion and may be the result of unstable family relationships and/or a lack of interpersonal relationship skills in adolescents. Both victimization and perpetration of interpersonal violence may be associated with recurrent patterns of violent involvement across relationships. However, intermittent violent behaviors may occur without previous exposures and may commence or cease at any point. In contrast, aggression and violence are a part of some adolescents' daily lives. Thus, relationship violence is a more general means of interpersonal relating, not only a tool of conflict resolution.

With the exception of those children who have experienced child maltreatment, the first encounter many adolescents have with aggression occurs via bullying from peers. Conceptually, bullying is a malicious and repetitive action that reinforces and establishes a power inequity between the "bullier" and the "bullied."[2] Inherent with the formation of more intimate relationships between youth

---

*Corresponding author.
E-mail address: vir2002@columbia.edu (V. I. Rickert).

Copyright © 2007 American Academy of Pediatrics. All rights reserved. ISSN 1934-4287

during adolescence is increased peer coercion. Coercion is an exploitative strategy that is used to exert power and manipulate the intended victim to the perpetrator's desire. Although the literature on adolescent coercion is sparse, it has been suggested that certain forms of coercion are common. Coercion can occur between friends (eg, pressure to smoke marijuana or date to enhance social status), or it can occur among intimate partners (eg, pressure to not use condoms). Bullying and coercion may be subsequently associated with all forms of relationship violence. As adolescents begin to develop intimate relationships and dating, violence between romantic partners can and does occur. In general, there are direct and indirect forms of violence; both are powerful and encompass actions that impair an adolescent's development as well as his or her health. Indirect forms of interpersonal violence include gossiping and its emotional effects, whereas direct forms of violence are associated with harm or threat of harm to body integrity. Relationship violence during adolescence is complex and continues to evolve as adolescents mature.

Understanding of violence is constrained by available research relative to sexual orientation and gender. That is, references to romantic partners are mainly limited to heterosexual pairings because of the lack of research on lesbian, gay, bisexual, and transgender (LGBT) youth. Unfortunately, LGBT populations' experiences relating to interpersonal violence have been acutely more salient than their successes in intimate and peer relationships. In addition, gender is usually reported in a binary fashion; there is a desperate need for more research that includes transgender and non–gender-conforming youth. Finally, adolescent boys are typically portrayed as the perpetrators of violence and generally as a gender that suffers few negative consequences. These young men's complex realities also merit additional research. We believe that research conducted with these populations will add insight and deepen our understanding of interpersonal violence among all youth.

BULLYING

As children transition from childhood to early adolescence, their methods for relating to peers continue to develop, and bullying perpetration and/or victimization may reach elevated levels. During childhood, bullying is typically expressed by verbal aggression such as name-calling, but it can also be expressed physically in actions such as pushing or hitting. Significant psychosocial and psychosomatic problems such as bed-wetting, stomachaches, and sleeping problems have been associated with the receipt of childhood bullying.[3] As might be expected, bullying is more common in early as compared with late adolescence[2,4-6] and may foreshadow violent or coercive behaviors among both those who bully and those who are victimized by this form of violence.[7]

Bullying is prevalent in middle and high schools, with 1 in 4 students reporting being bullied by indirect aggression (ie, yelling or spreading rumors).[2] Bullying peaks around ninth grade[2,8] and is associated with depression, low self-esteem,[4,9,10] sexual risk taking, alcohol consumption, suicide, and further victimization.[5,9,10] Some risk factors for bullying include poor school adjustment and poor academic achievement.[4] Depression and anxiety are both identified as risk factors for and outcomes of being bullied in early adolescence.[3]

Gender differences in bullying among friendships and acquaintances are evident. Young men report the use of verbal and physical bullying; in contrast, young women report almost exclusively verbal and indirect bullying.[2,8] Among older adolescent girls, bullying behaviors range from direct verbal assault using humor or sarcasm to indirect exclusionary behaviors such as giving nasty looks, ignoring or neglecting the person, or spreading rumors.[11]

The rate of bullying for students who identify or are perceived as LGBT is higher than that for their heterosexual peers.[5,9,10,12] In fact, perceived sexual orientation is often used as a springboard for bullying independent of sexual preference. Thus, it should not be surprising that bullying experiences were disproportionately more common outcomes for lesbian, gay, and bisexual youth in schools in which high levels of school victimization were present.[10] Transgender youth are also at an increased risk for verbal bullying. One study found that these students experienced as much as 26 verbal assaults per day.[13] Regardless of gender identity and sexual orientation, bullying victimization may result in confusion, pain, and, ultimately, victim retaliation through similar means of violence.[11]

Bullying has important health implications, with bullies being more likely to engage in health risk behaviors including cigarette smoking and alcohol use.[4] Middle school aggression has been linked with initiating intimate partner violence (IPV) later in life.[7] In addition, bullies have reported increased perpetration of sexual aggression and are more likely to sexually harass both same- and opposite-gender peers.[2]

SEXUAL HARASSMENT

Concurrent with increased awareness of their sexual attractions and sexuality, single-gender peer networks expand to mixed-gender networks; group dating begins in early to middle adolescence. It has been suggested by Pepler et al[2] that during this developmental transition, bullying tactics evolve to include sexual aggression. For example, a longitudinal study found bullying to be significantly associated with sexual harassment and relationship violence.[2]

Adolescent boys and girls capitalize on their vulnerable peers through the use of sexual harassment.[2,8] Sexual harassment usually takes place outside of a dating relationship. Examples include indirect harassment such as sexually oriented comments and gossip relating to sex as well as more direct actions including name-calling or rubbing or brushing against someone in a sexual manner.[2] It is important to remember that sexual harassment occurs between same- and opposite-gender peers.[2,4,8] It is interesting to note that sexual harassment seems to be most prevalent in the 10th grade, 1 year after the peak incidence of bullying.[2,8] Similar to bullying, sexual harassment decreases as adolescents age, adjust to new social environments, and hone their interpersonal relationship skills.[2]

Similar to bullying, gender differences in contexts and outcomes for sexual harassment persist. As boys and girls progress in adolescence and start developing romantic relationships, there is increasing emphasis on traditional gender roles, which may make certain adolescents especially vulnerable to sexual harassment.[14] For example, male adolescents who do not conform to traditional masculine roles may be targeted as a way of controlling social gender norms.[14] These instances of harassment for both the initiator and recipient set a deeply negative precedent for communicating in personal relationships.

COERCION

Generally, bullying and sexual harassment diminish with increasing age and social adjustment,[2,4,5] whereas coercive behaviors may occur in late adolescence because of inadequate relationship skills as well as a strategy to manipulate romantic partners and peers. There has been limited research on coercion among adolescents but a growing acknowledgment among adolescent health care providers of its occurrence and the need for screening. Similar to bullying, coercion is best expressed as a continuum of behaviors along several domains: emotional/verbal, controlling, physical, and sexual. Although coercion between peers occurs, most research conceptualizes coercion among romantic or sexual partners.

Adolescents may directly coerce romantic partners through verbal threats, controlling their behaviors by continuously checking on activities, and by the use of physical force. Verbal and physical coercion may be easily recognized by adolescents when compared with sexual coercion or controlling behaviors. With regards to sexual coercion, which influences and/or pressures a person to engage in unwanted sexual activities, behaviors may vary from taunting to unwanted touching to pressure to not use condoms or birth control. Nuanced with elements of social and sexual desire, adolescents may need help and support in recognizing and responding to sexual coercion, because boundaries for appropriate sexual behavior are still forming in late adolescence. More discrete or indirect coercion such as controlling time spent together or apart, emotional manipulation, and isolating behaviors may be even more subtle and difficult-to-identify forms of coercion. While adolescents develop closer affiliations with their friends and start engaging in romantic relations, the line between healthy communication and controlling actions should be highlighted. Research has suggested that physical violence is becoming less acceptable to partners and peers and that this shifting social norm results in increasing levels of psychological abuse.[15]

Overall, perceptions of coercion are often flexible and context specific. Therefore, how youth define sexual coercion must be considered. Qualitative research by Sears et al[15] among middle school students has suggested that context is very relevant in determining whether adolescents believe that a specific action or behavior is coercive. In addition, these researchers found significant differences according to gender in perception of abuse. Thus, coercion is multifaceted, and it is important to clearly communicate what constitutes coercion when speaking to adolescents.

RELATIONSHIP VIOLENCE

As adolescents begin dating in dyads, those youth who experienced previous difficulties forming intimate relationships and resolving conflict may persistently engage in violent interpersonal relationships.[2,7] However, this progression of violence is not obligatory or standard, and relationship violence may occur without previous experience and/or exposure to violence or, alternatively, may not happen at all. The term "relationship violence" refers to verbal, emotional, physical, or sexual violence that occurs among romantic and sexual partners. Synonymous with IPV and dating violence, relationship violence has the same serious connotation for adolescents as IPV does for adults. Similar to coercion, relationship violence may include controlling behaviors but evolves to include social isolation and more direct and repetitive verbal, emotional, physical, and sexual violence to end or resolve disputes between partners or as an inappropriate manifestation of anger. A recent longitudinal study of older Latino and white adolescents found that young men who perpetrated violence against peers or intimate partners were more likely to express forms of violence concurrently and in the future.[16] These findings support the theory that a common thread of violence in an adolescent's life is manifested in multiple ways and may be pervasive among family, peer, and intimate partner relationships.

Verbal and Physical Violence

Physical violence and verbal abuse are all too common in adolescent romantic relationships. Although not particular to this age cohort, the prevalence of these forms of aggression remains high. According to the 2005 national Youth Risk Behavior Survey, 36% of respondents had been part of a physical fight, and 9% were purposefully hit, slapped, or physically hurt by an intimate partner in the previous year.[17]

Research has indicated that physical aggression is often, although not always, interactive and reciprocal.[7,18] Contrary to the stereotype that a young woman is always the victim of dating violence, young women often perpetrate violence against their male partners. However, injuries sustained by young women are usually more severe than injuries sustained by young men.[19] The prevalent societal norm against males hitting or otherwise physically abusing females may be partially responsible for uneven disclosure rates between genders and simultaneously may explain increases in controlling behaviors as a form of relationship violence.[15]

Sexual Violence

Along with sexual initiation, a significant proportion of older adolescents may experience sexual violence as either a perpetrator or victim. Sexual violence is typically defined broadly to encapsulate the wide range of forceful and coercive strategies that may be used to obtain sex. Remember that "rape" is a legal term that is defined as nonconsensual sex, but it has significantly different interpretations depending on the authority (eg, federal, state, local) involved in prosecution. Developmentally, sexual violence as either a victim or perpetrator may be connected to a history of inappropriate behaviors and hurtful relationships, including child sexual abuse, although this trajectory may fluctuate.

As Table 1 demonstrates, prevalence estimates for sexual violence can vary widely depending on how the data were collected and measured. Prevalence data from crime-reporting agencies and national surveillance data generate lower point estimates. Crime reports rely entirely on victims disclosing the offense to legal authorities, which reduces the likelihood that most sexual victimization would be captured. National surveillance surveys, on the other hand, often use 1 or 2 items that require respondents to make a judgment call about the nature of the event that has occurred (eg, "Have you ever been sexually assaulted?"). A respondent may either not recognize that the victimization she or he experienced fits under that rubric or not wish to label the experience. In either case, the reported proportion of adolescents who experience that type of victimization will be reduced.

Research that does not use surveillance measurement strategies often use more standardized measures of relationship violence. At a minimum these studies will measure the occurrence of violence with several items that assess victimization or perpetration behaviorally. For example, instead of asking respondents to label an event, a question will be asked about whether a specific act has occurred (eg, "Has anyone ever touched your genitals without your consent?" versus "Have you ever been molested?"). Each methodology has its merits, especially for what it is attempting to achieve, but in the end, we are left with an extremely fragmented picture of sexual victimization. We have simultaneously an image of aberrant violence occurring among a minority of female youth and pervasive victimization that neglects neither gender nor race.

A study of urban young women between 14 and 23 years old who were attending

TABLE 1. Prevalence Estimates for Relationship Violence

Type of Report	Measured Indicators	Violence Proportion, %	Notable Information
National crime reports			
Bureau of Justice Statistics; National Crime Victimization Survey, 2005[21]	Rape, sexual assault, nonfatal IPV (physical assault)	Forcible rape (females), 12–15 y, 0.24; 16–19 y, 0.57; 20–24 y; nonfatal IPV (females, 2004), 12–15 y, 0.16; 16–19 y, 0.42; 20–24 y, 1.15	Because Bureau of Justice Statistics data are based on crimes reported to authorities, the proportion reported here is significantly less than what may be reported elsewhere; data are collected as an aggregate and then segmented by age group; adolescents are not specifically targeted for all age groups, reported rates of sexual victimization for women are at least 3 times greater than those for men; for 16- to 19-y-old women, the rate is ~7 times greater
Federal Bureau of Investigation Uniform Crime Reports, 2005[22]	Forcible rape	College/university women, 0.008; all women, 0.317	Forcible rape is defined by the Federal Bureau of Investigation as the carnal knowledge of a female forcibly and against her will; any nonphysical or nonforced crimes or male victimizations are not included; statistics provided indicate victimizations that were reported to authorities; in the case of colleges and universities, information sharing between the Federal Bureau of Investigation and campus administration happens voluntarily: forcible rape accounts for ~5% of all violent crime on college campuses and 7% nationwide, according to reported statistics

TABLE 1. Prevalence Estimates for Relationship Violence (Continued)

Type of Report	Measured Indicators	Violence Proportion, %	Notable Information
National survey data			
Youth Risk Behavior Surveillance, 2005[23]	Dating violence, forced sexual intercourse	Dating violence (females) 9.3, (males) 9.0; forced sexual intercourse (females) 10.8, (males) 4.2	Sexual violence is assessed from 1 item on the Youth Risk Behavior Surveillance questionnaire, which includes all forms such as date/acquaintance rape and child sexual abuse; the Youth Risk Behavior Surveillance survey does not distinguish between degrees of coercion or force; percentage of students reporting violence increased significantly for both forced sexual intercourse and dating violence between 9th and 12th grade
Finkelhor et al, Developmental Victims Survey, 2005[24]	Six sexual victimization categories with subcategories assigned for different perpetrators.	Sexual victimization (adolescents 13–17 y) 16.8; sexual assault (adolescents 13–17 y) 6.7	National cross-sectional sample of youth 2 to 17 y old; approximately half of the sample was ≥10; acquaintances account for 91% of all perpetrators; 86% of perpetrators were juveniles
Tjaden and Thoennes National Violence Against Women Survey, 1998[25]	Child sexual abuse, rape, stalking, physical violence	Lifetime prevalence of rape (male) 3.0, (female) 17.6; age at first time of rape (female) < 12 y, 21.6; 12–17 y, 32.4; 18–24 y, 29.4; >25 y, 16.6	National telephone survey involving random-digit dialing; two items assessed victimization; demographic comparisons between the sample and the population in general were made by using 1995 census data; this sample may similarly suffer from criticisms aimed at the census data (eg, under-representative of lower SES, minorities); females averaged ~3 acts of victimization per rape victim, whereas males averaged 1

an adolescent health clinic found that nearly one third experienced an unwanted sexual solicitation within the previous 12 months.[20] This ethnically diverse sample provided prevalence statistics that were significantly higher than any of those from the national data, which requires one to consider whether a significant victimization burden is being ignored on a national level. A longitudinal study that was conducted at rural junior high schools in North Carolina yielded similarly high prevalence statistics among a significantly younger cohort.[26] The probability that a young woman who had not been previously victimized would experience a form of sexual violence between 8th and 12th grades was 1 in 5. For dating violence, the probability for both young men and young women was also ~1 in 5.

RISK FACTORS

There is broad agreement on the risk factors associated with sexual assault, physical violence, verbal abuse, and coercion (Table 2). One element in particular remains significantly linked to victimization (regardless of race, gender, or socioeconomic status): previous exposure to or experience with violence. It is important to stress that violence is an act that victimizes the recipient, the perpetrator, and the witness jointly.[18]

With some exceptions,[6,16,18,26] most studies have suffered from the limitations of cross-sectional designs that do not allow for the determination of causality. Regardless of this fact, the temporal relationship between violence in the home and both perpetration and victimization later in life has been clearly established. Similarly, studies have found a strong link between physical abuse experienced during early adolescence and later perpetration of physical and sexual dating violence.[7,18]

HELP-SEEKING BEHAVIORS

Despite its high prevalence, most adolescents, regardless of whether they perpetrate violence or are a victim, do not seek help.[27-29] Those adolescents who do seek assistance often turn to family and friends before ever considering disclosing information to a clinician.[28] Young women, however, support screening for IPV and emphasize that the attitude and approach of a provider is important.[30] These data are critical. Screening to detect violent experiences represents an important public health strategy for overcoming the difficulty that adolescents may experience in attempting to disclose relationship violence.

SEQUELAE

Although reactions of adolescent victims may parallel adult responses, their specific developmental stage must be taken into account. Victimization experiences can lead to persistent negative effects on self-confidence and identity.

TABLE 2. Risk Factors for Violence and Sexual Assault Victimization

Physical and Verbal Violence and Coercion
  Females
    Exposure to family violence
    A history of abuse (sexual or other) or exposure to abuse
    Alcohol use among whites
    Depression
    Previous suicidal ideation
    Number of dating partners
    Having a friend who has been victimized by dating violence
    Engaging in unprotected sex without contraceptives
  Males
  Exposure to family violence
    A history of abuse (sexual or other) or exposure to abuse
    Alcohol use among whites
    Low self-esteem
    Lack of anger management skills
Sexual Assault
  Females
    Age: 16–24
    A history of abuse (sexual or other)
    Alcohol use among whites
    Early age of menarche
    Acceptance of rape myths
    Greater number of dating or sexual partners
  Sexually active peer group
    Dating relationship that includes verbal or physical abuse
  Males
    A history of abuse (sexual or other)
    Alcohol use among whites
    Acceptance of rape myths
    Homelessness
    Physical, cognitive, or psychiatric disability

Simultaneously with victimization the young person is discovering and navigating feelings of sexual arousal, autonomy, and intimacy.

Behavior after violence and aggression may range from denial to uncharacteristic and inappropriate behavior or, alternatively, self-isolation. Extra familial or peer attention may be needed but rejected, and relationships previously deemed important may suffer from neglect and withdrawal. The differentiation between expected independence from family during adolescence and more serious withdrawal from friends and activities in addition to parents is crucial, and the latter may suggest serious problems. Higher levels of depression and anxiety are associated with these negative experiences. After sexual assault by a romantic partner, appearance of symptoms of posttraumatic stress disorder are not uncommon within 1 year.[31]

In cases of sexual coercion, an adolescent may experience increased confusion and difficulty differentiating between healthy sexual pleasure and violence, especially if their first sexual experience was coerced or violent. In addition, higher incidences of risk-taking behaviors, such as unprotected sex or alcohol consumption, and harmful attitudes about sex may follow coercive experiences.[32] Early referral and multiple options for the adolescent may help increase their sense of self-autonomy and the likelihood that the teen will seek help.

CLINICAL IMPLICATIONS

The process of developing healthy interpersonal relationships is a major developmental task of adolescence, and clinicians have the opportunity to improve unhealthy relationships through screening and referral of their adolescent patients. Clinicians prevent violence by asking adolescent patients about their friendships and romantic relationships and clarifying that healthy relationships are free from all forms of interpersonal violence (Table 3). The method of inquiry and its presentation (ie, the language used in questions) should be considered carefully, because face-to-face questioning often yields lower levels of disclosure in comparison to self-administered screenings, even when they are not anonymous. Ensuring confidentiality and assisting adolescents who need help in leaving unhealthy relationships is critical. Screening should not be implemented in the clinical setting before appropriate referral systems are in place.

In early adolescence, it is critical to inquire about family and peer relationships as well as peer networks. Through conversation, the clinician needs to establish the character of these relationships to determine the level of attachment, support, and security. One method is to ask direct questions about relationships (eg, "Who do you rely on?" "What are your friends like?" "What do you like to do with your friends?"). If there are problems in these relationships, additional evaluation by a mental health profession would be warranted.

Once the clinician has established with reasonable certainty that family and peer relationships are appropriate, further querying about teasing (or being teased) in school or frequent problems/fights with friends or peers will alert the clinician to bullying behaviors. Follow-up questions can include concerns regarding school avoidance, previous exposure to violence, and fear of harm. Remember that it is important to identify both perpetrators and victims of bullying, because both are associated with later relationship violence. Interventions for both victims and perpetrators can include direct work with the school and individual therapy.

Direct questioning about unwanted sexual comments or touching can uncover sexual harassment, its frequency, and its severity. In the most extreme cases, alerting schools or reporting these situations (if the youth consents) can help the youth to get needed support and reaffirm that sexual harassment is unacceptable. For youth who are questioning their sexuality, sexual harassment can be partic-

TABLE 3. Developmentally Appropriate Questions About Intimate Relationships

Relationships and families
  Early
    Who do you talk to when you're upset?
    Have you ever witnessed violence in your home?
    Do you feel supported? By whom?
  Late
    How do you get along with your family?
Friendships: Same Sex and Opposite Sex
  Early
    Do you have a best friend?
    Where are your friends? In school or in the neighborhood?
  Late
    What do you do with your friends?
    Do you talk to your friends when you need advice or when you're upset?
    Do you have fights or disagreements with your friends?
    Do you trust your friends?
Romantic Relationships
  Early
    Do you have a crush on anyone?
  Late
    Tell me about your partner.
    What do you like about your partner?
    How does your partner treat you?
    Do you ever feel unsafe with your partner?
    Does your partner ever make you feel bad about yourself?
    Does your partner make you feel like a better person or bring you down?
Peer Groups
  Early
    Who do you spend time with?
  Late
    Do you care what your friends think about your partner?
    What do you do when you hang out with your friends?

ularly harmful, and it is important to screen these adolescents for depression and suicide.

Because coercion can occur in both peer and dating relationships, it is important to recognize any patterns of coercion. For example, the clinician can ask why a teen is engaging in certain risk behaviors such as drinking or using drugs and why they first started. Process questions can uncover the influence of peers or partners and identify the teen who is particularly vulnerable to coercive strategies.

When discussing relationships with older adolescents, balancing inquiries about positive and negative relationship characteristics provides the opportunity for adolescents to disclose important information. Questions that address how the partner treats them, what their arguments are about, who makes decisions regarding sex (particularly condom use), and direct questions about sexual force and physical violence are important. Asking these questions can underscore that violent behavior is not acceptable and that help can be sought.

As adolescents proceed through their development, they learn about and establish intimate ties through their relationships with family, friends, and, eventually, romantic partners. An adolescent's community of peers, romantic partners, family, and health care providers can all contribute to their development of healthy relational skills. Unfortunately, for some adolescents this process may be interspersed or interrupted with instances of violence and aggression. Clinicians who are equipped to recognize patterns of unhealthy relationships and offer resources when adolescents are at risk for poor outcomes can contribute to ensuring not only the present safety of their patients but also the future health of their intimate relationships. Adolescents want healthy intimate romantic and peer relationships; health care providers can assist them in developing the needed skills and support to help achieve those relationships.

REFERENCES

1. Raymond M, Catallozzi M, Lin AJ, Ryan O, Rickert VI. Development of intimate relationships in adolescence. *Adolesc Med.* 2007;18:449–459
2. Pepler DJ, Craig WM, Connolly JA, Yuile A, McMaster L, Jiang DP. A developmental perspective on bullying. *Aggress Behav.* 2006;32:376–384
3. Fekkes M, Pijpers FIM, Fredriks AM, Vogels T, Verloove-Vanhorick SP. Do bullied children get ill, or do ill children get bullied? A prospective cohort study on the relationship between bullying and health-related symptoms. *Pediatrics.* 2006;117:1568–1574
4. Nansel TR, Overpeck M, Pilla RS, Ruan WJ, Simons-Morton B, Scheidt P. Bullying behaviors among US youth: prevalence and association with psychosocial adjustment. *JAMA.* 2001;285: 2094–2100
5. Eisenberg ME, Aalsma MC. Bullying and peer victimization: position paper of the Society for Adolescent Medicine. *J Adolesc Health.* 2005;36:88–91
6. Pellegrini AD, Long JD. A longitudinal study of bullying, dominance, and victimization during the transition from primary school through secondary school. *Br J Dev Psychol.* 2002;20:259–280
7. O'Donnell L, Stueve A, Myint-U A, Duran R, Agronick G, Wilson-Simmons R. Middle school aggression and subsequent intimate partner physical violence. *J Youth Adolesc.* 2006;35:693–703
8. Craig WM, Pepler DP. Identifying and targeting risk for involvement in bullying and victimization. *Can J Psychiatry.* 2003;48:577–582
9. Goodenow C, Szalacha L, Westheimer K. School support groups, other school factors, and the safety of sexual minority adolescents. *Psychol Sch.* 2006;43:573–589
10. Bontempo DE, D'Augelli AR. Effects of at-school victimization and sexual orientation on lesbian, gay, or bisexual youths' health risk behavior. *J Adolesc Health.* 2002;30:364–374
11. James VH, Owens LD. "They turned around like I wasn't there": an analysis of teenage girls' letters about their peer conflicts. *Sch Psychol Int.* 2005;26:71–88
12. Berlan ED, Corliss HL, Field AE, Goodman E, Austin B. Sexual orientation and bullying in adolescents. *J Adolesc Health.* 2007;40:S28
13. Kimmel MS, Mahler M. Adolescent masculinity, homophobia, and violence: random school shootings, 1982-2001. *Am Behav Sci.* 2003;46:1439–1458
14. Fineran S, Bolen RM. Risk factors for peer sexual harassment in schools. *J Interpers Violence.* 2006;21:1169–1190

15. Sears HA, Byers ES, Whelan JJ, Saint-Pierre M. "If it hurts you, then it is not a joke": adolescents' ideas about girls' and boys' use and experience of abusive behavior in dating relationships. *J Interpers Violence.* 2006;21:1191–1207
16. Ozer EJ, Tschann JM, Pasch LA, Flores E. Violence perpetration across peers and partner relationships: co-occurrence and longitudinal patterns among adolescents. *J Adolesc Health.* 2004;34:64–71
17. Eaton DK, Kann L, Kinchen S, et al. Youth risk behavior surveillance: United States, 2005. *J Sch Health.* 2006;76:353–372
18. Arriaga XB, Foshee VA. Adolescent dating violence: adolescents follow in their friends', or their parents', footsteps? *J Interpers Violence.* 2004;19:162–184
19. Jackson SM, Cram F, Seymour FW. Violence and sexual coercion in high school students' dating relationships. *J Fam Violence.* 2000;15:23–36
20. Rickert VI, Wiemann CM, Vaughan RD, White JW. Rates and risk factors for sexual violence among an ethnically diverse sample of adolescents. *Arch Pediatr Adolesc Med.* 2004;158:1132–1139
21. Catalano SM. Criminal Victimization, 2005. *Bureau of Justice Statistics Bulletin.* Washington, DC: US Department of Justice; 2006 September. Publication NCJ 214644
22. Federal Bureau of Investigation. *Crime in the United States.* Washington DC: Federal Bureau of Investigation; 2005. Available at: http://www.fbi.gov/ucr/05cius/. Accessed November 9, 2007
23. Centers for Disease Control and Prevention. Youth Risk Behavior Surveillance—United States, 2005. Surveillance Surmmaries, 2006 June 9. MMWR 2006;55 (No. SS-5)
24. Finkelhor D, Ormrod R, Turner H, Hamby SL. The victimization of children and youth: a comprehensive, national survey. *Child Maltreat.* 2005;10:5–25
25. Tjaden P, Thoennes N. *Full Report of the Prevalence, Incidence, and Consequences of Violence Against Women: Findings From the National Violence Against Women Survey.* Washington, DC: National Institute of Justice, Office of Justice Program, US Dept of Justice, and Centers for Disease Control and Prevention; 2000. Publication NCCJ 183781
26. Foshee VA, Benefield TS, Ennett ST, Bauman KE, Suchindran C. Longitudinal predictors of serious physical and sexual dating violence victimization during adolescence. *Prev Med.* 2004; 39:1007–1016
27. Ashley OS, Foshee VA. Adolescent help-seeking for dating violence: prevalence, sociodemographic correlates, and sources of help. *J Adolesc Health.* 2005;36:25–31
28. Ocampo BW, Shelley GA, Jaycox LH. Latino teens talk about help seeking and help giving in relation to dating violence. *Violence Against Women.* 2007;13:172–189
29. Rickert VI, Wiemann CM, Vaughan RD. Disclosure of date/acquaintance rape: who reports and when. *J Pediatr Adolesc Gynecol.* 2005;18:17–24
30. Zeitler MS, Paine AD, Breitbart V, et al. Attitudes about intimate partner violence screening among an ethnically diverse sample of young women. *J Adolesc Health.* 2006;39:119.e1–119.e8
31. Rickert VI, Ryan O, Chacko M. Sexual violence and victimization. In: Neinstein LS, Gordon C, Katzman D, Woods ER, Rosen D, eds. *Adolescent Healthcare: A Practical Guide.* 5th ed. Philadelphia, PA: Lippincott, Williams & Wilkins; 2007: In press
32. Diaz A, Simantov E, Rickert VI. Effect of abuse on health: results of a national survey. *Arch Pediatr Adolesc Med.* 2002;156:811–817

Office-Based Interventions to Promote Healthy Sexual Behavior

Jennifer Christner, MD[a], Pamela Davis, MD[b], David S. Rosen, MD, MPH[a],*

[a]*Division of Child Behavioral Health and* [b]*General Pediatrics, Department of Pediatrics, University of Michigan Medical School, 1500 E. Medical Center Drive, Ann Arbor, MI 48109*

Addressing the needs of teenagers efficiently in a busy practice can often seem like a daunting challenge. The adolescent often requires more time, with attention to confidentiality and other issues that are not required by younger patients. Promoting healthy sexuality and sexual behavior encompasses a broad variety of topics that need to be discussed sensitively and at a developmentally appropriate level for the teenager in an office setting that is adolescent-friendly. The American Medical Association, in their guidelines for adolescent preventive services, specifically state that discussing sexuality with both teens and parents is an essential task of the physician as part of preventive health visits.[1] With teens, this discussion should occur at least on an annual basis. However, an experienced clinician can use a variety of clinical encounters as opportunities for private conversations once the parent has left the examination room. The American Medical Association also recommends that sexuality be discussed with parents at least 3 times, once each during early, middle, and late adolescence.[1]

OFFICE DESIGN, STAFF, AND POLICIES

To most effectively meet the needs of adolescent patients, several steps must be taken even before the patient is actually seen. The ability to discuss healthy sexuality with a teenager begins with having an office and staff that are teen-friendly. A separate waiting area and examination rooms that are designed specifically with adolescent needs in mind sends a strong welcoming message to teenagers. Such a setup would include having age-appropriate educational and recreational reading materials available as well as examination rooms that are already outfitted with equipment and supplies for pelvic examinations. Although an appealing environment sets the stage, it is essential that the staff, including front-desk staff, are specifically trained and knowledgeable regarding consent

---

*Corresponding author.
E-mail address: rosends@med.umich.edu (D. S. Rosen).

and confidentiality issues that pertain to teens. Teens are more likely to confide sensitive issues once they know that confidentiality is assured.[2] A recent study demonstrated that 47% of girls under 18 years of age would stop using sexual health care services if mandatory parental notification of services were implemented.[3] Many primary care pediatric offices are not prepared to deliver confidential services to adolescents, but minors actually have rights to such care for a range of health issues.[4] Each state has its own laws that deal with consent and confidentiality regarding the diagnosis and treatment of sexually transmitted infections (STIs), prenatal care, pregnancy, abortion, and mental health issues. Several excellent resources exist that allow review of the laws of individual states[5] (Table 1).

It can be very helpful to use clinical staff meetings to review the laws of one's particular state. Then, setting aside a portion of each staff meeting for both clinical and nonclinical personnel to discuss parent telephone calls or other concerns that relate to teen care is helpful. For example, staff members may have personal or religious concerns regarding premarital sex and/or the use of emergency contraception. Although it may be beneficial to explore these issues before hiring, what is important is how each employee will make patients feel when they call or arrive. A nurse who refuses to administer injectable contraception or call in emergency contraception will impose tasks on other staff and may impede office workflow if not addressed proactively. However, with regular meetings, confusion or personal biases in dealing with these and similar issues can be aired and resolved while at the same time reinforcing expectations for the delivery of care. It might also be useful to note that the American Academy of Pediatrics, the American College of Obstetrics and Gynecology, the American Medical Association, and the Society of Adolescent Medicine all agree that teenagers should

Table 1
Resources

Legal issues
   Alan Guttmacher Institute: www.guttmacher.org
   Center for Adolescent Health & the Law: www.adolescenthealthlaw.org
Free patient handouts/brochures
   CDC: www.cdc.gov/std (fact sheets/posters on STIs)
   US Department of Health and Human Services and SAMHSA: http://ncadi.samhsa.gov (fact sheets/brochures on drugs and alcohol)
Immunization resources
   CDC: www.cdc.gov/std/HPV/STDFact-HPV.htm
   Immunization Action Coalition: www.immunize.org
Web sites for teens and parents
   American Academy of Pediatrics: www.aap.org/stress (teens can build their own stress management plan)
   YoungWomensHealth.org: www.youngwomenshealth.org (an award-winning Web site for teen girls sponsored by Children's Hospital Boston that features health guides, quizzes, chats, and more)

be guaranteed confidentiality when reproductive health care is delivered.[1,6] Developing specific office policies and having these position statements readily available is valuable when training new staff. The American College of Obstetrics and Gynecology has developed a sample telephone script and written confidentiality agreements for both patients and parents and a sample written office policy that addresses confidentially concerns that parents may have.[7]

Confidentially of records is very important. Teens may reveal things to their provider that they do not want their parents to know. Be certain that there is an understanding of state laws, including their rights under the Health Insurance Portability and Accountability Act (HIPAA), and that an office policy has been developed to clarify that medical charts do not leave the office unless they are reviewed for content. If state law permits, confidential parts of charts may be excluded. At a minimum, the way in which confidential information is disclosed must be managed.

There should also be training regarding how to schedule appointments for teenagers. Some staff may think that a parent needs to call for an appointment and will refuse to schedule with an adolescent, so it is essential to discuss with staff the policy regarding teens calling to schedule their own appointments. If a teenager calls for an appointment, it is likely that the adolescent perceives an urgent need and, therefore, should be accommodated as rapidly as possible.

Teen appointments can be very time consuming, but there are ways to maximize efficiency. Examine scheduling guidelines for ways to maximize the time spent with teen patients. Seeing teens frequently can decrease lengthy visits. Limit discussions to 1 or 2 high-priority topics at each visit and schedule return visits as necessary. Stress a willingness to address other issues but that each issue deserves adequate time, which may require additional visits.

It can be difficult to balance the need for teen autonomy and confidentiality with the value of parent support and education, but it is important to make sure that both parents and teenagers are fully aware of and understand these policies. It can be very helpful to begin early (at age 9 or 10 years) to initially spend some limited time alone with the preteen, thus allowing both patients and parents time to adjust to the idea of private time. At a new-patient visit with the teen and the parent in the room, it is often helpful to review office policies regarding confidentiality. Seeing both the adolescent and parent together at the beginning of the visit provides the clinician with valuable information and allows the parent/guardian the opportunity to verbalize and then process any concerns. Giving parents reassurance that they will be brought back to the room at the end of the visit can often help allay anxiety/hesitation when they are asked to leave. Walking out of the room with the parent may allow the parent additional time to express other questions or concerns. Once back in the room with the teenager, emphasize the confidential nature of questions and discussion, but also review situations in which disclosure would need to occur (eg, life-threatening risks or situations). Encourage patients to involve their parent(s) in discussions about sexuality and offer, if appropriate, to facilitate the conversation. Before the parent's return to the room, negotiate with the adolescent exactly what topics will be discussed with the parent and in what detail. Careful attention to points of confidentiality previously agreed upon will engender trust in the physician.

ADDRESSING ADOLESCENT SEXUALITY IN THE OFFICE SETTING

Adolescents

Each adolescent should receive developmentally appropriate counseling regarding sexuality and sexual behavior, including discussion of abstinence, the choice to become sexually active, role playing to delay becoming sexually active, contraception, and prevention of and screening for STIs. The nature and content of counseling must be developmentally appropriate and will be determined by age, cognitive skills, pubertal development, emotional and social maturity, risks, strengths, and protective factors. The history obtained should also cover the potential of possible sexual abuse and violence, which are among the topics discussed in this issue of *AM:STARs*.

Preadolescents and early adolescents (~8–13 years of age) are concrete thinkers and do not fully understand how their behaviors relate to their health. Counseling should be clear and direct, and involving parents will allow reinforcement of counseling points. Discussion regarding physical/emotional changes, changing relationships with parents, and emerging sexual thoughts can be addressed with these patients. Examination of the external genitalia throughout childhood and preadolescence helps children become more comfortable with their own body and can normalize and set the stage for less uncomfortable future examinations during adolescence.

Middle adolescents (~14–17 years of age) are characterized by further physical development and social/emotional changes with the beginning of abstract thinking. Capable of more complex, logical thinking, teens in this age group typically make more decisions that may affect both their health and health care. Experimentation with risky behaviors often occurs in this population, because puberty is nearly complete. These patients are becoming more private about their bodies and sexuality, which makes it more difficult for them to raise related issues with health care providers. Teens often appreciate clinicians broaching these sensitive topics in a nonjudgmental, respectful manner. These teens want accurate information regarding sexuality but find it difficult to inquire; thus, they often get information (much of it inaccurate or incomplete) from their peers and/or the media, as discussed by Brown et al[8] in this issue. Myths surrounding pregnancy and STI transmission abound in this group. Discussion topics should include responsible decision-making, the range of sexual expression, and beliefs regarding premarital sex. Role-playing exercises that deal with sexual refusal skills and coercion can be very useful.

Late adolescents (~18–24 years of age) have a more sophisticated understanding of how their behavior affects their health than do younger patients. This understanding, coupled with abstract reasoning skills, allows them to present and consider health decisions in the broad context of future goals. Providing adolescents with hypothetical dilemmas in which they can openly explore their feelings and weigh conflicting options can help them to further develop mature decision-making skills. Even so, it is estimated that approximately one third of adolescents and, thus, adults do not make the transition to abstract reasoning.[9] Parenting style and role modeling may play a large role in this development stage. By choosing role playing as the mainstay of risk-reduction counseling, the physician may help promote the development of abstract reasoning in the course of providing sexuality education.

These discussions are often confined to yearly preventive services visits or to the annual pelvic examination. However, any acute-care visit should be considered to be a potential opportunity for addressing these issues with teens. Although teens report that their health care provider is one of their primary sources of information regarding health topics, ~50% of teens report being too embarrassed to discuss sexuality with a primary care provider.[10] One study indicated that topics of sexual activity and prevention of pregnancy were discussed in only 30% of primary care visits, although 58% of the teens thought that it should be discussed.[10]

Clinicians

To the extent possible, it is valuable for young patients to see the same clinician throughout their adolescence. Developing rapport and comfort with the physician can enable open discussion regarding sexuality (and other) issues. If a teen is not regularly seen by the same physician and only presents for acute complaints, an effort should be made to introduce additional screening for health risk behaviors and a follow-up appointment arranged to discuss specific concerns in more detail. Open-ended questions such as, "Have you discussed sex with your friends?" and "What do they think about it?" can be a way of opening the conversation. It is important for discussions to be interactive, nonjudgmental, and supportive. For example, "This is an age at which many teenagers start to think about sexual relationships" can normalize the adolescent's thoughts. Discussing issues such as acne, weight management, or sleep disturbance (common teen complaints) during an acute visit may help the patient bring up even more sensitive questions. The realization that the physician may be genuinely concerned about the adolescent's comfort and well-being can facilitate communication. Whatever the approach, it is essential for clinicians themselves to be comfortable when talking to patients about sexuality and to communicate in common, informal language.

Family

Patient confidentiality regarding sexuality is both critical and a conundrum. For many adolescents, privacy is clearly important. However, parental involvement is also critical in making good decisions, especially for younger teens. Parental disapproval of sexual intercourse results in report of lower occurrence of sexual intercourse and increased abstinence.[11] Teens consistently report that they want to discuss their sexuality with their parents. They look to their parents for both health information and input into defining and clarifying their values. Teens are more reluctant, however, to talk with parents if they perceive a knowledge deficit or parental discomfort. Explaining the rationale for confidentiality while continuing to actively involve the parents in health care visits can help parents become educated and more aware of important issues, thus facilitating the discussion with their teens regarding sexuality concerns.

Peers

Although teens can be reluctant to address sexuality with their parents or physician, discussion with peers occurs often. As a result, peers represent the primary source of health information for many adolescents. Therefore, ask teens about information that they may have obtained from their peer group ("Are any of your friends using birth control?" "What adverse effects have you heard about?"). In doing so, the physician may trigger a discussion that addresses unspoken concerns. Teens often feel more comfortable asking questions when they are with a member of their peer group. Encourage them to return with a friend if they prefer. Another option is to schedule a group counseling session for teens to discuss issues of menstruation and sexuality. These approaches not only provide education for the patient but also create opportunities to educate other teens. Providing each adolescent with age-appropriate written information can be invaluable in educating others because it may encourage them to distribute the educational material to other teens. As an example, discussing with a teen that pelvic examinations are no longer required to obtain contraception may result in that teen becoming an educational "ambassador" to other teens.[12]

Addressing sexual orientation is an important part of promoting sexual health and is discussed in more depth elsewhere in this volume. Teens may experiment with both same- and opposite-gender encounters before self-identifying or being comfortable with expressing their sexual orientation. Primary care providers often do not ask about these experiences or may not create a climate in which teens are comfortable raising these issues.[13] An American Academy of Pediatrics policy statement that addressed sexuality recommended that all youth (including nonheterosexual youth) be provided with a medical office that is safe, supportive, and nonjudgmental. Pediatricians are encouraged to make their office a place in which teens feel comfortable discussing these topics by assuring confidentiality, using gender-neutral language, and providing comprehensive health care and counseling. One must also recognize the unique problems that nonheterosexual youth may face with issues such as body image, depression, and risky behaviors.[14] Additional discussion of this very important topic is offered by Spigarelli[15] (in this issue).

ADHERENCE

Adolescents often have difficulty adhering to any medical regimen, which can affect their sexual health. Having a consistent approach to these issues can make them more manageable. First, ensure that no mental health issues are interfering with care. A teen who is depressed will have difficulty focusing on being healthy and adhering to treatment recommendations. Make certain that the teen understands and agrees with the treatment plan. Adequate information and education are essential for good adherence. Also, there are a variety of logistic issues that may interfere with treatment. Can the teen or his or her parents afford the prescribed medication? Does the teen have access to transportation to appear for scheduled appointments?

Once these practical issues have been addressed, work with patients to better understand how they view the pros and cons of adherence. Teens may find aspects of their treatment regimens unreasonable (eg, taking medication at school or tolerating particular adverse effects). Can changes be made to address these barriers that do not compromise the goals of treatment? Negotiate the treatment plan if necessary as long as the negotiated plan does not jeopardize safety. Finally, help teens consider how their current health will affect their achieving their current and future goals.

MEDICAL NEEDS OF THE SEXUALLY ACTIVE PATIENT

Pelvic Examination

The first pelvic examination is usually met with great anxiety. Fortunately, new guidelines allow deferral of the first Papanicolaou test in a healthy teen until 3 years after sexual activity begins or until 21 years of age.[16] The availability of noninvasive STI testing via self-vaginal swab or first-void urine specimen has allowed appropriate screening for STIs without requiring a pelvic examination. Setting aside a separate visit for the initial pelvic examination gives the clinician additional time to better attend to patients' anxiety. Education about the examination, the instruments, and the testing materials to be used is helpful. During the visit, several techniques can be used to minimize discomfort and anxiety. Make certain to use an appropriately sized speculum (for most adolescent patients, a Huffman or Pederson speculum). Assure the patient that she can stop the examination at any time. During the examination, talking through each step and each touch is essential. Pausing during the examination is often needed. Occasionally, the adolescent will test the examiner's promise to stop the examination, but once she is reassured, the examination can proceed. If an adolescent is extremely anxious, has significant pain with the examination, or has pain with light touch of the external genitalia, then establishing the reasons for her concerns (including the possibility of sexual abuse) must be pursued once the examination is completed and she is again dressed.

Testing for and Treating STIs

The adolescent and young-adult population maintains the highest STI rate in the United States. While representing only 25% of the sexually active population, 15- to 24-year-olds account for nearly half of all STI diagnoses each year.[17] For this reason, all sexually active adolescents should be screened yearly for STIs and, on the basis of recent Centers for Disease Control and Prevention (CDC) guidelines, HIV.[18] More frequent rescreening for *Chlamydia trachomatis* should be considered, particularly for those who previously tested positive, have new symptoms, have a history of a new partner, and/or report inconsistent condom use.[19]

Screening for asymptomatic infections in adolescents may not be understood. Concrete thinking makes it difficult for some patients to understand the importance of testing when they feel "fine." It may also be difficult for some adolescents to accept that their partner may not be monogamous or has had previous partners. Last, because some teens engage in "only" oral sex, they do not consider themselves to be sexually active. However, screening should be considered so as not to miss genital infections in these at-risk patients.[20] Asking detailed questions regarding level of involvement in intimacy (eg, kissing, heavy petting, oral sex, use of sexual devices) can elicit risk-factor information about STI transmission. It is important that the physician take adequate time to explore these issues with the adolescent.

Fortunately, newer, noninvasive testing methods for both men and women permit screening that patients find less aversive. Urine-based testing for both *Neisseria gonorrhea* and *C trachomatis* is available and is nearly as sensitive as traditional urethral and cervical swab methods. Urine testing requires a "dirty catch"; the patient should not have urinated 1 hour before specimen collection or cleaned the genitalia before urinating. Self-obtained vaginal swabs may be collected for both *N gonorrhea* and *C trachomatis* testing.

After the testing is complete, how should positive test results be communicated? Before testing, it is critical to create a plan for reporting results to the patient. Sending a written report to a teenager's home may inadvertently breech confidentiality and significantly damage the patient's trust in the provider. Obtaining a telephone number at which a message can be left confidentially is optimal. If this is not possible, it is best to have the adolescent schedule a return visit to discuss results.

When a patient with a positive test result returns to the clinic for treatment, the importance of informing and treating his or her partner should be discussed. If the patient is uncomfortable discussing the results with a previous partner, anonymous reporting can be offered. With this method, the patient can give the nursing staff the name and contact information of the partner. This partner will be contacted and informed that someone with whom they had sexual contact tested positive for an STI and that they also need treatment. Expedited partner treatment (giving the patient a prescription for the treatment of his or her partner's STI) has been shown to decrease the recurrence rate of STIs.[21,22] However, expedited partner treatment is controversial, because it does not allow for risk-reduction counseling and screening for other STIs in the partners; expedited partner treatment is specifically prohibited in some US states.[23]

Immunizations

Excellent reviews on adolescent vaccination are available.[24,25] Two vaccines are essential for promoting sexual health. The hepatitis B vaccine has been universally recommended by the American Academy of Pediatrics since 1992. Although most teens will have completed this series in infancy, it is essential to review adolescents' health records to ensure that they have been fully immunized, because infection through sexual partners is a common route of transmission. There is no need to restart the series even if the doses have been separated by several years time.

Although the hepatitis B vaccine has been widely accepted, vaccine against human papilloma virus (HPV) is new and has been the subject of some controversy. For the HPV vaccine to be fully effective, it must be given before the onset of sexually activity. Several studies have demonstrated that the physician's strong recommendation of the vaccine may be the most effective strategy to encourage parents to vaccinate their daughters.[26] One should approach HPV vaccination in a matter-of-fact manner. For example, "Brittany is due for her first dose of HPV today. This vaccine can prevent her from getting cervical cancer, which is the second most common cause of cancer in reproductive organs in women." If the parent resists HPV vaccination, take the time to understand why and offer information regarding the vaccine. Many parents are simply unfamiliar with HPV and are concerned about the age at which the vaccine should be given. However, provider recommendations have a strong influence on the parent's ultimate decision.[27] Therefore, reinforce the medical benefits of vaccine cancer prevention. Direct the parents to reputable information (eg, from the CDC's Web site) for more help with making or validating their decision.

Addressing Contraception in the Office Setting

One of the biggest challenges in addressing adolescent sexuality is contraception. As a population, most adolescents do not seek contraceptive services until they have been sexually active for 6 to 12 months. The delay in seeking contraception is a result of inadequate or inaccurate information, concerns about resources, concerns about confidentiality, ambivalence regarding pregnancy, and anxiety surrounding the pelvic examination.[28] As a result, 50% of adolescent girls will become pregnant within 6 months of initiating sexual intercourse.[29]

Often, adolescents will present for abdominal pain or upper respiratory infection symptoms only to ask about birth control as you are closing the visit. It is difficult to provide adequate counseling during a 15-minute acute-care visit on a busy day. Laying the groundwork during preventive health visits can be helpful. Having a nurse who has been trained in educating adolescents about contraceptive choices (just as some are educated about asthma treatment) can allow for comprehensive counseling while protecting physician time. Even in the absence of previous counseling, contraception can usually be prescribed in a relatively brief visit. Question the adolescent about her last menstrual cycle, her most recent episode of unprotected intercourse, her personal and family history of thromboembolic disease, and her smoking history. Obtaining blood pressure and a urine pregnancy test are adequate, quick screening tests. A pelvic examination is not routinely required. Providing the patient with a contraceptive method before leaving the office is ideal, which may mean keeping a small supply of medication in the office or clinic. Offering injectable medroxyprogesterone (Depo Provera) for interim contraception is effective protection while providing sexually active young women additional time to consider their choice of methods. If use of a contraceptive cannot begin on the day of the visit, ask for a confidential telephone number to enable follow-up. Once a contraceptive method has been selected, the level of adherence should receive careful attention.

For 3 decades, oral contraceptive pills (OCPs) have been the most commonly used method of hormonal birth control. OCP failure rates vary according to age, race, socioeconomic status, and marital status. Most sources have quoted a 3% to 8% failure rate for all women, whereas in some populations, the failure rate is as high as 18%. Inconsistent pill-taking has been identified as the primary source for OCP failure. Overall, 16% of users do not follow the recommended OCP schedule. Studies of female adolescents have shown that 20% to 30% miss a pill every month.[30] Using traditional methods of taking the medication at bedtime or first thing in the morning may not work with adolescents' inconsistent schedules. The use of longer-term methods such as the transdermal patch (OrthoEvra), vaginal ring (NuvaRing), injectable medroxyprogesterone (Depo Provera), or the intrauterine device can increase compliance. For the clinician, it is important to provide the adolescent with options, outline relevant risks, and facilitate an individualized decision that best meets her specific needs and preferences.

Although no studies have revealed teratogenicity with any hormonal contraception, traditional guidelines have suggested waiting for a normal menstrual cycle before starting hormonal contraception. This typically causes a delay in achieving adequate protection. Newer "quick-start" or "immediate-start" strategies have shown better compliance as well as decreased pregnancy rates.[31,32] Young women who have been sexually active but have a negative urine pregnancy test result should be counseled regarding the risk of an early, undetected pregnancy. Emergency contraception can be offered if appropriate and the birth control method is started immediately. Patients should be counseled regarding the need for a repeat pregnancy test if they do not have a normal cycle within the next 4 weeks. With quick start of any method, including medroxyprogesterone, the adolescent will need additional contraceptive protection (abstinence, condoms, or spermicides) for at least the next 7 days.

Parental and/or partner knowledge and support affect contraceptive compliance. Although many adolescents do not want their parents informed about their contraceptive choices, engaging both parties (eg, framing the need for contraception related to premenstrual syndrome, dysmenorrhea, or treatment of acne) can promote constructive discussion in a less threatening environment. Parental support for a birth control method increases adolescent adherence.[33,34] Partner knowledge and support for a contraceptive method can also increase adherence. Discussion of sexuality with young men often centers on STI prevention and condom use. However, male adolescents were more likely to report that their partners used a hormonal method of birth control throughout the previous year after contraception education.[35] For older, sexually active adolescents, scheduling a visit with her partner can be helpful.

Social myths and concerns about real or imagined adverse effects also play a significant role in successful contraceptive use. Concerns about weight gain, moodiness, increased risk of cancer, and future fertility are widespread in the community. Adverse effects are the primary reason for discontinuation of any hormonal contraceptive method. Even so, the adolescent may be uncomfortable raising these concerns in the clinical setting. The clinician, therefore, must raise these issues in an age-appropriate manner to dispel myths and improve adherence. Asking the adolescent what she has heard about various contraceptive methods can be a way of obtaining information about unspoken fears. Focused counseling regarding potential adverse effects, the decrease in adverse effects with time, and effective management of adverse effects can make the young woman less apprehensive and more willing to continue contraceptive use.

The volume of new information given in a contraceptive counseling visit can be overwhelming. The sensitive nature of the information may also make it difficult for the adolescent to attend to the information presented. Giving written information can be an effective means of improving education and allows additional review in private or with an adolescent's partner or parents.

Emergency Contraception

In addition to discussing conventional contraceptive regimens with the adolescent, it is important to address emergency contraception. The original Yuzpe regimen consists of 2 combined estrogen and progestin doses that are taken 12 hours apart. Unfortunately, this method has resulted in frequent nausea and vomiting. The newer levonorgestrel-only method (Plan B) has a similar efficacy rate with fewer adverse effects.[36] Although Plan B may be taken up to 120 hours after an unprotected sexual contact, efficacy ranging from 60% to 94% is highest with decreased time to first dose. New data have shown that taking both tablets at 1 time is just as effective as the 12-hour dosing strategy.[37] Plan B is now available without a prescription for young women who are 18 years and older. Explaining the use of emergency contraception and advance prescribing enables young women to obtain prompt treatment without waiting to be seen in the office or clinic. Although advanced prescribing of emergency contraception results in a four- to sixfold increase in its use, it has not been accompanied by a decrease in hormonal contraception use or an increase in unprotected sexual activity.[38]

CONCLUSIONS

Providing care to adolescents is both challenging and rewarding, and this is no more true than when addressing sexual health. Preparation of the office and office staff is helpful in maximizing efficiency and avoiding conflict. A clear policy on confidentiality, scheduling, and release of records also eliminates confusion and helps provide optimal care to the patients. Once the foundation has been established, the challenge is to balance active parental involvement with adolescents' emerging autonomy, being willing to tackle touchy and sometimes controversial counseling issues in a nonjudgmental manner, and ensuring that the patients' sexual health needs are met.

REFERENCES

1. American Medical Association. *AMA Guidelines for Adolescent Preventive Services (GAPS): Recommendations and Rationale.* Baltimore, MD: Williams and Wilkins; 1994
2. Anderson SL, Schaechter J, Brosco JP. Adolescent patients and their confidentiality: staying within legal bounds. *Contemp Pediatr.* 2005;22:54–64
3. Reddy DM, Fleming R, Swain C. Effect of mandatory parental notification on adolescent girls' use of sexual health care services. *JAMA.* 2002;288:710–714
4. Akinbami LJ, Gandhi H, Cheng TL. Availability of adolescent health services and confidentiality in primary care practices. *Pediatrics.* 2003;111:394–401
5. English A, Morreale M, Hersh C, Stinnett A. *State Minor Consent Statutes: A Summary.* 2nd ed. Chapel Hill, NC: Center for Adolescent Health and the Law; 2001
6. Sigman G, Silber TJ, English A, et al. Confidential health care for adolescents: position paper for the Society of Adolescent Medicine. *J Adolesc Health.* 1997;21:408–415
7. Physicians for Reproductive Choice and Health. Adolescent Reproductive Health Education Project: Education Project Curriculum. New York, NY: Physicians for Reproductive Choice; 2006

8. Brown JD, Strasburger VC. From Calvin Klein to Paris Hilton and MySpace: adolescents, sex, and the media. *Adolesc Med.* 2007;18:484–507
9. Woolfolk AE, McCune-Nicolich L. *Educational Psychology for Teachers.* 2nd ed. Englewood Cliffs, NJ: Prentice-Hall; 1984
10. Ackard DM, Meumark-Sztainer D. Health care information sources for adolescents: age and gender differences on use, concerns, and needs. *J Adolesc Health.* 2001;29:170–176
11. Dittus PJ, Jaccard J. Adolescents' perceptions of maternal disapproval of sex. *J Adolesc Health.* 2000;26:268–278
12. Mulchahey KM. Practical approaches to prescribing contraception in the office setting. *Adolesc Med Clin.* 2005;16:665–674
13. Allen LB, Glicken AD, Beach RK, Naylor KE. Adolescent health care experience of gay, lesbian, and bisexual young adults. *J Adolesc Health.* 1998;23:212–220
14. Frankowski BL; American Academy of Pediatrics, Committee on Adolescence. Sexual orientation and adolescents. *Pediatrics.* 2004;113:1827–1832
15. Spigarelli MG. Adolescent sexual orientation. *Adolesc Med.* 2007;18:508–518
16. Saslow D, Runowicz CD, et al. American Cancer Society guidelines for the early detection of cervical neoplasia and cancer. *CA Cancer J Clin.* 2002;52:342–362
17. Weinstock H, Berman S, Cates W Jr. Sexually transmitted diseases among American youth: incidence and prevalence estimates, 2000. *Perspect Sex Reprod Health.* 2004;36:6–10
18. Centers for Discase Control and Prevention. Sexually transmitted disease treatment guidelines, 2006. Available at www.cdc.gov/std/treatment/#g2006. Accessed August 1, 2007
19. Hu D, Hook EW. Screening for *Chlamydia trachomatis* in women 15–29 years of age: a cost-effectiveness analysis [published correction appears in *Ann Intern Med.* 2004;141:744]. *Ann Intern Med.* 2004;141:501–513
20. Sanders SA, Reinisch JM. Would you say you "had sex" if...? *JAMA.* 1999;281:275–277
21. Golden MR, Whittington WLH, Handsfield HH, et al. Effect of expedited treatment of sex partners on recurrent or persistent gonorrhea or chlamydial infection. *N Engl J Med.* 2005;352:676–685
22. Centers for Disease Control and Prevention. Expedited partner therapy in the management of sexually transmitted diseases. Available at: www.cdc.gov/std/treatment/EPTFinalReport2006.pdf. Accessed May 1, 2006
23. Centers for Disease Control and Prevention. Legal status of expedited partner therapy (EPT). Available at: www.cdc.gov/std/ept/legal/default.htm. Accessed May 2006
24. Middleman AB, Rosenthal SL, Rickert VI, et al. Adolescent immunizations: a position paper of the Society of Adolescent Medicine. *J Adolesc Health.* 2006;38:321–327
25. Rupp RE, Rosenthal SL. New immunization strategies for adolescent patients. *Adolesc Health Update.* 2006;19(1):1–8
26. Moscicki, AB. Impact of HPV infection in adolescent populations. *J Adolesc Health.* 2005;37(6 suppl):S3–S9
27. Olshen E, Woods ER, Austin SB, Luskin M, Bauchner H. Parental acceptance of the human papilloma virus vaccine. *J Adolesc Health.* 2005;37:248–251
28. Louis Harris and Associates, Inc. *American Teens Speak; Sex, Myths, TV, and Birth Control.* New York, NY: Planned Parenthood Federation of America; 1986
29. Feldman E. Contraceptive care for the adolescent. *Prim Care.* 2006;33:405–431
30. Hillard PJ. Oral contraception noncompliance: the extent of the problem. *Adv Contracept.* 1992;8(suppl 1):13–20
31. Westhoff C, Kerns J, Morroni C, Cushman LF, Tiezzi L, Murphy PA. Quick start: a novel oral contraceptive initiation method. *Contraception.* 2002;79:322–329
32. Rickert JI, Tiezzi L, Leon J, Lipshutz J, Vaughan RD, Westhoff C. Depo now: preventing unintended pregnancies among adolescents. *J Adolesc Health.* 2006;38:96
33. Jaccard J, Dittus PJ. Adolescents' perceptions of maternal approval of birth control and sexual risk behavior. *Am J Public Health.* 2000;90:1426–1430
34. Miller BC. Family influences on adolescent sexual and contraceptive behavior. *J Sex Res.* 2002;39:22–26

35. Danielson R, Marcy S, Plunkett A, Wiest W, Greenlick MR. Reproductive health counseling for young men: what does it do? *Fam Plann Perspect.* 1990;22:115–121
36. Hansen LB, Saseen JJ, Teal SB. Levonorgestrel-only dosing strategies for emergency contraception. *Pharmacotherapy.* 2007;27:278–284
37. von Hertzen H, Piaggio G, Ding J, et al. Low dose mifepristone and two regimens of levonorgestrel for emergency contraception: a WHO multicentre randomized trial. *Lancet.* 2002;360:1803–1810
38. Conard LE, Gold MA. Emergency contraceptive pills: a review of the recent literature. *Curr Opin Obstet Gynecol.* 2004;16:389–395

Approaches to Adolescent Sexuality Education

Mary A. Ott, MD[*,a], John S. Santelli, MD, MPH[b]

[a]Section of Adolescent Medicine, Department of Pediatrics, Indiana University School of Medicine, 410 West 10th Street, HS1001, Indianapolis, IN 46202, USA

[b]Heilbrunn Department of Population and Family Health, Mailman School of Public Health, Columbia University, 60 Haven Avenue, New York, NY 10032, USA

Developing a healthy sexuality is a key developmental task for adolescents. Healthy sexuality includes, "sexual development, reproductive health, and such characteristics as the ability to develop and maintain meaningful interpersonal relationships, appreciate one's own body; interact with both genders in respectful and appropriate ways; and express affection, love, and intimacy in ways consistent with one's own values."[1]

In recent years, adolescent sexuality has moved from being an issue of the health and well-being of adolescents to being a politically volatile and divisive topic. Nowhere is this shift more relevant to adolescent health and well-being than in the area of sexuality education. The purpose of this article is to provide background on adolescent sexual behavior, to review the current sexuality education policy landscape, to examine data that support different educational approaches, and to discuss specific concerns with federal support of abstinence-only education.

SEXUAL AND REPRODUCTIVE BEHAVIOR

Sexuality is a normal part of development. It becomes a public health concern when sexual behavior poses a health risk to oneself or others (eg, through unintended pregnancy or sexually transmitted infections [STIs]). This stands in contrast to other adolescent health risk behaviors and/or conditions such use of tobacco and obesity, which are unhealthy under any circumstances. The need to recognize sexuality as a normal and healthy part of development makes sexuality education more complex than other types of education that deal with behaviors that affect health.

---

*Corresponding author.
E-mail address: maott@iupui.edu (M. A. Ott).

Copyright © 2007 American Academy of Pediatrics. All rights reserved. ISSN 1934-4287

Knowledge of sexual behaviors, both during adolescence and across the life span, provides a necessary context for understanding adolescent sexuality. Few American adults abstain from sexual intercourse until marriage, and most initiate sexual intercourse during their adolescent years. After declining between 1991 and 2001 (from 54% to 46%), sexual experience among US high school students from 2001 to 2005 remained stable at 46% to 47%.[2] In the United States, there has been an 8- to 10-year gap between the median age of first intercourse (17 years) and first marriage (25 years for women and 27 for men).[3,4] An analysis of 4 cycles of the National Survey of Family Growth found that by age 20, 77% of Americans reported sexual experience (nearly all of it premarital sex), and by age 44, 99% reported sexual experience (95% premarital sex).[5]

Unintended pregnancy and STIs are significant causes of adolescent morbidity. Although pregnancy rates have declined, the United States still leads the developed world in adolescent (ages 15–19) birth rates, with 42 births per 1000 women in 2004. By comparison, adolescents in the United Kingdom had 27 births per 1000 women, in Italy 7 births per 1000 women, and in the Netherlands 5 births per 1000 women.[6] Most adolescent pregnancies (82%) are unintended,[7] and >28% of these pregnancies end in abortion.[8] Of importance to sexuality education, a recent analysis of the 1995 and 2002 National Surveys of Family Growth showed that 86% of the decline in adolescent pregnancy was a result of improved contraceptive use (less nonuse, increased use of condoms and hormonal methods, and increased use of dual methods); 14% was a result of declines in sexual behavior.[9]

For STIs, young people aged 15 to 24 account for almost half of the 19 million new infections each year. Young women have the highest age-specific rates of gonorrhea and chlamydia, and large racial and ethnic disparities persist in disease prevalence.[10]

DEFINITIONS

Abstinence

Adolescents demonstrate a complex and often nuanced view of abstinence and sex. Although refraining from vaginal intercourse is generally considered "abstinence," other sexual behaviors (eg, touching, kissing, mutual masturbation, oral sex, and anal sex) may or may not be considered as such.[11,12] Adolescents frequently frame abstinence from a values or religious perspective, using descriptors such as, "making a commitment" or "my religion says...."[13,14] Unlike adults, recent data suggested that adolescents do not view abstinence as a binary state (having sex/not having sex) but, rather, view abstinence as a stage in the normal trajectory of sexual development.[13]

Abstinence-Only Education

For this review, we labeled sex-education programs as "abstinence-only education" if the program adheres to federal requirements for abstinence-education funding. Federal guidance specifies that programs must have as their "exclusive purpose" the promotion of abstinence outside of marriage, requires programs to follow an 8-point definition of abstinence-only education (see Table 1), and specifies that programs may not in any way advocate contraceptive use or discuss contraceptive methods or condoms except to emphasize their failure rates.[15] These programs are also known as "abstinence-until-marriage" programs and have been marketed recently as "relationship education."

Comprehensive Education

Many definitions of comprehensive sexuality education exist. For the purposes of this review, we defined comprehensive sexuality education as an educational program that provides medically accurate information on contraception, condom use, and other safer sexual behaviors, in addition to abstinence.

Advocates of comprehensive sexuality education describe the goals of comprehensive sexuality education broadly: (1) to develop in adolescents a positive view of sexuality; (2) to provide information to take care of adolescents' sexual health; (3) to help adolescents acquire skills to make decisions about relationships and sexuality; and (4) to provide an opportunity for adolescents to question, explore, and assess their own and their community's attitudes about gender and sexuality.[16] Informational needs include accurate and developmentally appropriate

Table 1
Federal 8-point definition of abstinence education

Under §510 of Title V of the Social Security Act, abstinence education is defined as an educational or motivational program that
    has, as its exclusive purpose, teaching the social, psychological, and health gains to be realized by abstaining from sexual activity;
    teaches abstinence from sexual activity outside marriage as the expected standard for all school-aged children;
    teaches that abstinence from sexual activity is the only certain way to avoid out-of-wedlock pregnancy, STIs, and other associated health problems;
    teaches that a mutually faithful monogamous relationship in the context of marriage is the expected standard of human sexual activity;
    teaches that sexual activity outside of the context of marriage is likely to have harmful psychological and physical effects;
    teaches that bearing children out-of-wedlock is likely to have harmful consequences for the child, the child's parents, and society;
    teaches young people how to reject sexual advances and how alcohol and drug use increases vulnerability to sexual advances; and
    teaches the importance of attaining self-sufficiency before engaging in sexual activity

information about growth and development, reproduction and anatomy, masturbation, family life, pregnancy and childbirth, parenthood, sexual response, sexual orientation, contraception, abortion, sexual abuse, and HIV/AIDS and other STIs.[16] Skills include communication; decision-making; assertiveness; peer refusal; the capacity to create and maintain caring, supportive, noncoercive, and mutually pleasurable intimate and sexual relationships; and the use of contraceptives.[16] This focus on skills is to help young people exercise responsibility regarding sexual relationships by addressing such issues as abstinence, contraception, and the healthy expression of sexuality.[16]

SEX-EDUCATION LANDSCAPE

Public Support for Abstinence and Comprehensive Sexuality Education

Public-opinion surveys have demonstrated broad public support for comprehensive sexuality education, with abstinence as a key component of that education. A nationally representative survey of American adults showed that 81% believed sex education that teaches both abstinence and contraception to be effective, whereas only 39% believed abstinence-only education to be effective.[17] The same survey found that 51% of the adults opposed abstinence-only education, whereas only 10% opposed teaching contraception and condom use. Among parents of North Carolina public school students, 91% believed that sex education should be taught in school, with 98% rating transmission and prevention of STIs/HIV as important, 91% rating abstinence as important, 93% rating how to talk with a partner about birth control as important, and 89% rating effectiveness and failure rates of birth control as important.[18] A third national survey showed that most parents and adolescents do not perceive education that stresses abstinence and also provides information about contraception as presenting a mixed message, and the clear majority of the adults (73%) and adolescents (56%) wished that adolescents were getting more information about both abstinence and contraception rather than either alone.[19]

Federal Support for Sexuality Education

For fiscal year 2007, the federal government provided $176 million for abstinence-only education through Title V, §510 of the Social Security Act, community-based abstinence education (CBAE) projects, and the Adolescent Family Life Act program (www.nonewmoney.org/history.html). The bulk of this funding goes to CBAE programs, which bypass state government approval processes and make grants directly to community-based organizations, including faith-based organizations. Although the 2008 debates on the reauthorization of Title V and CBAE programs will shift federal dollars, the approximate amount that goes to abstinence-only education will likely stay the same. No designated federal funding stream exists for comprehensive sexuality education.

Erosion of Comprehensive Sexuality Education

Several studies have documented the erosion of comprehensive sexuality education coincident with the rising emphasis on abstinence as the sole option for adolescents.[20,21] The most recent data compared 1995 to 2002 and showed a decline in young women who reported receiving education about contraception (87% to 70%), coupled with an increase in abstinence-only education (8% to 21%), which resulted in fewer of these women receiving formal instruction about both abstinence and birth control methods (84% to 65%).[20]

Abstinence-only approaches have also influenced family planning and HIV-prevention programs nationally and internationally. In fiscal year 2004, the Office of Population Affairs announced that program priorities for Title X grantees would include a focus on extramarital abstinence education and counseling.[22] The Government Accountability Office (GAO), which is the investigative arm of the US Congress, criticized US foreign policy support for abstinence-only education and found that requiring funds to be spent on abstinence-only approaches limits developing nations' "efforts to design prevention programs that are integrated and responsive to local prevention needs."[23]

IMPORTANT ISSUES IN SEX EDUCATION

The 3 most important and timely aspects of a science-based approach are (1) program evaluation and the use of effective programs, (2) the medical and scientific accuracy of program content, and (3) ethical and human rights issues in sexuality education.

Program Effectiveness

Sexuality education, like much education policy, has moved toward science-based approaches. This has been spearheaded by the Centers for Disease Control and Prevention (CDC) with cooperative agreements with 3 national organizations: Advocates for Youth, the National Campaign to Prevent Teen Pregnancy, and the Healthy Teen Network. A key aspect of science-based approaches is the use of process and outcome evaluation of the implemented program and modifying that approach on the basis of results. A science-based program is one that research has shown to be effective in changing sexual behavior. A promising program is one that has not been formally evaluated but has most of the characteristics of programs that have been shown to be effective.[24]

Comprehensive Sexuality Programs

Comprehensive sexuality programs have been shown to change adolescent sexual behavior. Several systematic reviews of program evaluations have documented changes such as delaying the onset of coitus, decreasing coital frequency, and increasing condom use.[25–30,33,34]

Abstinence-Only Programs

In contrast, abstinence-only programs have not been shown to change the adolescent sexual behaviors listed above. A federally funded evaluation of Title V programs that was conducted by an independent research organization,[31] 5 systematic reviews,[26,27,32–34] and analyses of nationally representative longitudinal surveys of health behavior[35] demonstrated that abstinence-only programs are ineffective and may cause harm.

The most important single report is Mathematica Policy Research, Inc's final report on the impact of 4 Title V, §510 abstinence-education programs.[31] Authorized by the US Congress and using a rigorous randomized, controlled trial study design, investigators examined the impact on sexual behaviors among 2057 adolescents 4 years after participation in 1 of 4 carefully chosen and implemented Title V abstinence-only programs or a community-standard control. The report described no differences in sexual abstinence or condom use between those in the abstinence-only program group and those in the control group. A concern was that youth in the intervention group were significantly less likely to report that condoms were effective in preventing HIV and other STIs. This finding is consistent with the emphasis in abstinence-only curricula on teaching about the failure rates for condoms, as required by federal program guidance.[36]

Three recent peer-reviewed systematic reviews joined 2 older systematic reviews in concluding that there is no evidence that abstinence-only programs delay the initiation of sexual intercourse.[26,27,32–34] These 5 reviews used similar scientific criteria for selecting program evaluations, including use of experimental or quasi-experimental design and the use of sexual behavior outcomes to demonstrate efficacy.

The findings from the above-mentioned randomized trial and systematic reviews are supported by a longitudinal analysis of adolescents who took virginity pledges in the National Longitudinal Study of Adolescent Health.[35,37] At the 6-year follow-up, 88% of participating young adults who reported taking virginity pledges as adolescents had initiated vaginal intercourse before marriage, and the prevalence of STIs (chlamydia, gonorrhea, and trichomoniasis) was similar among pledgers and nonpledgers.[35] Moreover, when pledgers did initiate intercourse, many failed to protect themselves by using condoms and were less likely to be tested for STIs. These data suggest that, although abstinence is theoretically 100% effective, in typical use the effectiveness of abstinence as a means of preventing pregnancy and STIs is extremely low.[36]

Medical and Scientific Accuracy

Fueled by recent congressional and GAO reports, concerns about the medical accuracy of sex education have come to the forefront. From a scientific and public health standpoint, it is essential that information provided through sexual and reproductive health education be medically and scientifically accurate. Medical accuracy can be defined as:

Information relevant to informed decision-making based on the weight of scientific evidence, consistent with generally recognized scientific theory, conducted under accepted scientific methods, published in peer-reviewed journals, and recognized as accurate, objective, and complete by mainstream professional organizations such as AMA [American Medical Association], ACOG [American College of Obstetricians and Gynecologists], APHA [American Public Health Association] and AAP [American Academy of Pediatrics], government agencies such as the Centers for Disease Control and Prevention (CDC), the Food and Drug Administration (FDA) and the National Institutes of Health (NIH), and scientific advisory groups such as the Institute of Medicine and the Advisory Committee on Immunization Practices. The deliberate withholding of information that is needed to protect life and health (and therefore relevant to informed decision-making) should be considered medically inaccurate.[39]

Advocates for comprehensive sexuality programs call for complete and accurate medical information on reproduction, contraception, and STIs.[16] However, individual comprehensive sexuality education programs may or may not be medically accurate. An important community role for pediatricians is to be able to advise and educate schools and community groups on medical accuracy.

For abstinence-only education, both federal abstinence-only funding guidelines and the manner in which funds are administered have raised serious concerns about medical accuracy. In the fall of 2006, the GAO issued 2 reports on the federal programs that promote abstinence, both of which faulted the programs on the issue of medical accuracy.[40,41] In the first report, the GAO concluded that the federal statutory requirement to include medically accurate information on condom effectiveness would apply to abstinence-education materials prepared and used by federal grant recipients.[40] The GAO further concluded that guidelines requiring abstinence-only programs to emphasize failure rates were potentially out of compliance.[40] The second GAO report faulted the US Department of Health and Human Services for not reviewing abstinence grantees' educational materials for scientific accuracy and not requiring grantees to review their own materials for scientific accuracy.[41]

As expected when the very guidance requires medical inaccuracy,[15] many abstinence-only curricula have been found to be medically inaccurate. A content review of abstinence-only curricula conducted by the minority staff of the Committee on Government Reform of the US House of Representatives found that 11 of the 13 commonly used curricula contained false, misleading, or distorted information about condoms, contraceptive use, abortion, and the risks of sexual activity.[42] The American Civil Liberties Union and other advocacy groups have publicly questioned the federal government's support for abstinence education on grounds of medical accuracy.[43] A review of 3 curricula commonly used by federal abstinence-funding grantees identified both explicitly and implicitly conveyed messages that condoms fail to provide protection against STIs.[44] Misrepresentations included the use of data from poorly designed studies and the exclusion or distortion of data from better-designed studies; routinely presenting information out of context; selectively reporting data; and drawing unsupported conclusions that go beyond the scope of the medical literature.[44]

Ethical Standards

Here we switch the focus from individual programs to broader policies. The current US government approach of focusing on abstinence-only education raises serious ethical and human rights concerns. Although abstinence is often presented as the moral choice for adolescents, abstinence-only policies have been identified as unethical because they require programs to deliberately withhold or distort potentially life-saving information.[45–47] Access to complete and accurate HIV/AIDS and sexual health information has been recognized as a basic human right, because complete and accurate health information is essential to realizing the highest attainable standard of health.[48,49] International treaties and human rights statements support an adolescent's right to accurate and complete sexual health information.[50,51] Such human rights thinking suggests that governments have an obligation to provide accurate information to their citizens and avoid the provision of misinformation. This obligation extends to government-funded health education and health care services such as funding for sexuality education and reproductive health. Withholding information on contraception to induce adolescents to be abstinent is inherently coercive (and ineffective, as documented above). It violates the principle of beneficence (to do good and avoid harm), because it may cause an adolescent to use ineffective (or no) protection against pregnancy and STIs. Withholding information on contraception additionally violates the principle of "respect for persons" and the commonly accepted practice of informed consent, because it requires the health educator to withhold information from a patient to influence their health care choices.[52]

PROFESSIONAL CONSENSUS STATEMENTS AND POSITION PAPERS

Mainstream medical professional organizations, including the American Academy of Pediatrics, the Society for Adolescent Medicine, the American Medical Association, the American College of Obstetricians and Gynecologists, and the American Public Health Association, oppose abstinence-only education and endorse comprehensive sexuality education that includes both abstinence and accurate information about contraception, human sexuality, and STIs.[46,47,53–56] The most comprehensive of these position papers is the Society for Adolescent Medicine's position paper and accompanying review article.[38,46] This pair of articles described the importance of scientific rigor as the cornerstone for policy and programmatic decisions, as well as the troublesome ethical issues raised by deliberately withholding or distorting potentially life-saving sexual health information.

SELECTING AND ADAPTING A COMPREHENSIVE SEXUALITY PROGRAM FOR A COMMUNITY

As noted above, the field of sexuality education has moved toward the use of science-based approaches. The gold standard is to use a proven or promising curricula, as defined by the CDC.[24] Proven programs have been evaluated and shown to change sexual behaviors by using a rigorous experimental (individual students are randomly assigned to a program or comparison group) or quasi-experimental (classrooms, schools, or similar groups are randomly assigned to a program or comparison group) evaluation design. Sources for proven effective programs can be found through the CDC, the National Campaign to Prevent Teen Pregnancy, Advocates for Youth, Sociometrics, Inc, and others (see Table 2). Promising programs have not yet been evaluated but contain many of the characteristics of effective programs.[57] These characteristics include, but are not limited to (1) developing theory-based, developmentally appropriate education programs that are sensitive to local needs, (2) connecting program elements to behavior to goals using logic models, (3) offering curricula that focus on risk and protective factors, clearly specified behaviors, and overall public health goals (eg, reducing unintended pregnancy), and (4) using instructionally sound and culturally appropriate educational activities and (5) are implementing the curricula with fidelity.[57] Specific guidelines for adapting programs have been compiled by the National Campaign to Prevent Teen Pregnancy and the Healthy Teen Network, in conjunction with the CDC (eg, see Putting What Works to Work by the National Campaign to Prevent Teen Pregnancy).[57,58]

Table 2
Resources for science-based programs

CDC: Adolescent reproductive health—promoting science-based approaches
    www.cdc.gov/reproductivehealth/AdolescentReproHealth/ScienceApproach.htm
Advocates for Youth: Programs that work to prevent teen pregnancy, HIV, and sexually
    transmitted infections in the United States and developing countries
    www.advocatesforyouth.org/programsthatwork/index.htm
Healthy Teen Network: Science-based approaches
    www.healthyteennetwork.org/index.asp?Type=B_LIST&SEC={84D38731-0591-41B6-90AF-03593EF836BA}
ETR, Inc: Resource center for adolescent pregnancy prevention
    www.etr.org/recapp/programs/index.htm
National Campaign to Prevent Teen Pregnancy: Putting What Works to Work
    www.teenpregnancy.org/works/default.asp
Sociometrics, Inc: Program archive on sexuality, health, and adolescence
    www.socio.com/pasha.htm
WHO (international programs): Special Programme of Research, Development and Research
    Training in Human Reproduction
    www.who.int/reproductive-health/hrp/index.htm

ROLE OF THE PEDIATRICIAN

Pediatricians are in a unique position to advocate for and advise communities and schools on comprehensive sexuality education programs, specifically

1. advocating for comprehensive sexuality education as the most effective approach to adolescent pregnancy and STI;
2. advising on the selection of science-based proven and promising programs;
3. insisting on the medical accuracy of information (including opposing curricula and approaches that deliberately withhold information on contraception and STIs); and
4. reframing the moral debate to make it clear that the provision of medically accurate and comprehensive information is the ethical choice.

REFERENCES

1. Sexuality Information and Education Council of the United States. Position statements on human sexuality, sexual health and sexuality education and information 1995–96. *SIECUS Rep.* 1996; 24(3):21–23
2. Eaton DK, Kann L, Kinchen S, et al. Youth Risk Behavior Surveillance: United States, 2005. *MMWR Surveill Summ.* 2006;55(5):1–108
3. Abma JC, Martinez GM, Mosher WD, Dawson BS. Teenagers in the United States: sexual activity, contraceptive use, and childbearing, 2002. *Vital Health Stat 23.* 2004;(24):1–48
4. Fields J. *America's Families and Living Arrangements: 2003.* Washington, DC: US Census Bureau; 2004
5. Finer LB. Trends in premarital sex in the United States, 1954–2003. *Public Health Rep.* 2007;122:73–78
6. United Nations Statistics Division. Table 11: live-birth rates by age of mother and urban/rural residence—latest available year, 1995–2004. Available at: http://unstats.un.org/unsd/demographic/products/dyb/DYB2004/Table11.pdf. Accessed May 21, 2007
7. Finer LB, Henshaw SK. Disparities in rates of unintended pregnancy in the United States, 1994 and 2001. *Perspect Sex Reprod Health.* 2006;38:90–96
8. The Guttmacher Institute. *US Teenage Pregnancy Statistics: National and State Trends and Trends by Race and Ethnicity.* New York, NY: Guttmacher Institute; 2006
9. Santelli JS, Lindberg LD, Finer LB, Singh S. Explaining recent declines in adolescent pregnancy in the United States: the contribution of abstinence and improved contraceptive use. *Am J Public Health.* 2007;97:150–156
10. Centers for Disease Control and Prevention, Division of STD Prevention. *Trends in Reportable Sexually Transmitted Diseases in the United States, 2005.* Atlanta, GA: US Department of Health and Human Services; 2006
11. Schuster MA, Bell RM, Kanouse DE. The sexual practices of adolescent virgins: genital sexual activities of high school students who have never had vaginal intercourse. *Am J Public Health.* 1996;86:1570–1576
12. Sanders SA, Reinisch JM. Would you say you "had sex" if? *JAMA.* 1999;281:275–277
13. Ott MA, Pfeiffer EJ, Fortenberry JD. Perceptions of sexual abstinence among high-risk early and middle adolescents. *J Adolesc Health.* 2006;39:192–198
14. Goodson P, Suther S, Pruitt BE, Wilson K. Defining abstinence: views of directors, instructors, and participants in abstinence-only-until-marriage programs in Texas. *J Sch Health.* 2003;73: 91–96
15. US Department of Health and Human Services, Administration for Children and Families. Community-based abstinence education program, funding opportunity number HHS-2007-ACF-

ACYF-AE-0099. Available at: www.acf.hhs.gov/grants/open/HHS-2007-ACF-ACYF-AE-0099.html. Accessed May 21, 2007
16. National Guidelines Task Force. *Guidelines for Comprehensive Sexuality Education, Kindergarten Through 12th Grade.* 3rd ed. New York, NY: Sexuality Information and Education Council of the United States; 2004
17. Bleakley A, Hennessy M, Fishbein M. Public opinion on sex education in US schools. *Arch Pediatr Adolesc Med.* 2006;160:1151–1156
18. Ito KE, Gizlice Z, Owen-O'Dowd J, Foust E, Leone PA, Miller WC. Parent opinion of sexuality education in a state with mandated abstinence education: does policy match parental preference? *J Adolesc Health.* 2006;39:634–641
19. Albert B. *With One Voice 2007: America's Adults and Teens Sound off About Teen Pregnancy.* Washington, DC: National Campaign to Prevent Teen Pregnancy; 2007
20. Lindberg LD, Santelli JS, Singh S. Changes in formal sex education: 1995–2002. *Perspect Sex Reprod Health.* 2006;38:182–189
21. Darroch JE, Landry DJ, Singh S. Changing emphases in sexuality education in U.S. public secondary schools, 1988–1999. *Fam Plann Perspect.* 2000;32:204–211, 265
22. Dailard C. Title X program announcement articulates new priorities for nation's family planning program. *Guttmacher Rep Public Policy.* 2003;6(5):13
23. US Government Accountability Office. Global health: spending requirement presents challenges for allocating prevention funding under the President's emergency plan for AIDS relief. Report GAO-06-395. Available at: www.gao.gov/new.items/d06395.pdf. Accessed August 21, 2006
24. Centers for Disease Control and Prevention. Adolescent reproductive health: promoting science based approaches. Available at: www.cdc.gov/reproductivehealth/AdolescentReproHealth/DefineScienceApproach.htm. Accessed August 21, 2007
25. Centers for Disease Control and Prevention, HIV/AIDS Prevention Research Synthesis Project. *Compendium of HIV Prevention Interventions With Evidence of Effectiveness.* Atlanta, GA: Centers for Disease Control and Prevention; 1999
26. Kirby DB, Laris BA, Rolleri LA. Sex and HIV education programs: their impact on sexual behaviors of young people throughout the world. *J Adolesc Health.* 2007;40:206–217
27. Kirby D. *Emerging Answers: Research Findings on Programs to Reduce Teen Pregnancy.* Washington, DC: National Campaign to Prevent Teen Pregnancy; 2001
28. National Campaign to Prevent Teen Pregnancy. *What Works: Curriculum-Based Programs That Prevent Teen Pregnancy.* Washington, DC: National Campaign to Prevent Teen Pregnancy. Available at: www.teenpregnancy.org/resources/reading/pdf/What_Works.pdf. Accessed November 7, 2007
29. Advocates for Youth. *Science and Success: Sex Education and Other Programs That Work to Prevent Teen Pregnancy, HIV and Sexually Transmitted Diseases.* Washington, DC: Advocates for Youth; 2003
30. Advocates for Youth. *Science and Success: Supplement I—Additional Sex Education and Other Programs That Work to Prevent Teen Pregnancy, HIV & Sexually Transmitted Infections.* Washington, DC: Advocates for Youth; 2006
31. Trenholm C, Devaney B, Fortson K, Quay L, Wheeler J, Clark M. *Impacts of Four Title V, Section 510 Abstinence Education Programs, Final Report.* Princeton, NJ: Mathematica Policy Research, Inc; 2007
32. Manlove J, Romano-Papillo A, Ikramullah E. *Not Yet: Programs to Delay First Sex Among Teens.* Washington, DC: National Campaign to Prevent Teen Pregnancy; 2004
33. Kirby D. Emerging Answers 2007: Research Findings on Programs to Reduce Teen Pregnancy and Sexually Transmitted Infections. Washington, DC: National Campaign to Prevent Teen and Unintended Pregnancy; 2007.
34. Underhill K, Montgomery P, Operario D. Sexual abstinence only programmes to prevent HIV infection in high income countries: systematic review. *Bmj,* 2000,335:248-259
35. Brückner H, Bearman P. After the promise: the STD consequences of adolescent virginity pledges. *J Adolesc Health.* 2005;36:271–278

36. US Department of Health and Human Services, Administration for Children and Families. Community-based abstinence education program, funding opportunity number HHS-2006-ACF-ACYF-AE-0099. Available at: www.acf.hhs.gov/grants/pdf/HHS-2006-ACF-ACYF-AE-0099.pdf. Accessed May 21, 2007
37. Bearman PS, Brueckner H. Promising the Future: virginity pledges and first intercourse. *Am J Sociol.* 2001;106:859–912
38. Santelli J, Ott MA, Lyon M, Rogers J, Summers D, Schleifer R. Abstinence and abstinence-only education: a review of U.S. policies and programs. *J Adolesc Health.* 2006;38:72–81
39. Santelli JS. Medical accuracy in sexuality education: ideology and the scientific process. *Am J Public Health.* 2007; In press
40. US Government Accountability Office. Abstinence education: applicability of section 317P of the Public Health Service Act. Available at: www.gao.gov/decisions/other/308128.pdf. Accessed October 15, 2007
41. US Government Accountability Office. Abstinence Education: Efforts to Assess the Accuracy and Effectiveness of Federally Funded Programs. Available at: www.gao.gov/new.items/d0787.pdf. Accessed October 15, 2007
42. US House of Representatives, Committee on Government Reform-Minority Staff. The content of federally funded abstinence-only education programs. Available at: http://oversight.house.gov/documents/20041201102153-50247.pdf. Accessed October 15, 2007
43. Kaiser Family Foundation. Daily HIV/AIDS report: politics and policy: HHS should enforce federal law that abstinence education programs teach 'medically accurate' information, ACLU letter says. Available at: www.kaisernetwork.org/daily_reports/rep_index.cfm?hint=1&DR_ID=44570. Accessed May 21, 2007
44. Santelli JS. Declaration of John S. Santelli, M.D., M.P.H. Available at: www.aclu.org/images/asset_upload_file220_29486.pdf. Accessed August 30, 2007
45. Human Rights Watch. *The Philippines: Unprotected Sex, Condoms, and the Human Right to Health.* New York, NY: Human Rights Watch; 2004
46. Santelli J, Ott MA, Lyon M, Rogers J, Summers D. Abstinence-only education policies and programs: a position paper of the Society for Adolescent Medicine. *J Adolesc Health.* 2006;38: 83–87
47. American Public Health Association. Abstinence and U.S. abstinence-only education policies: ethical and human rights concerns. Available at: www.apha.org/advocacy/policy/policysearch/default.htm?id=1334. Accessed October 15, 2007
48. Freedman LP. Censorship and manipulation of reproductive health information. In: Coliver S, ed. *The Right to Know: Human Rights and Access to Reproductive Health Information.* Philadelphia, PA: University of Pennsylvania Press; 1995:1–37
49. Coliver S. The right to information necessary for reproductive health and choice under international law. In: Coliver S, ed. *The Right to Know: Human Rights and Access to Reproductive Health Information.* Philadelphia, PA: University of Pennsylvania Press; 1995:38–82
50. United Nations, Population Information Network. A/CONF.171/13: Report of the International Conference on Population and Development (Cairo, September 5-13, 1994) (94/10/18). Available at: www.un.org/popin/icpd/conference/offeng/poa.html. Accessed October 15, 2007
51. Committee on the Rights of the Child. HIV/AIDS and the rights of the children. General Comment No. 3 (2003 A). Available at: www.unhchr.ch/tbs/doc.nsf/(symbol)/CRC.GC.2003.3.En?OpenDocument. Accessed May 21, 2007
52. US Department of Health. Protection of human subjects: Belmont report—notice of report for public comment. *Fed Regist.* 1979;44:23191–23197
53. American Academy of Pediatrics, Committee on Psychosocial Aspects of Child and Family Health and Committee on Adolescence. Sexuality education for children and adolescents. *Pediatrics.* 2001;108:498–502
54. American Medical Association. H-170.968: sexuality education, abstinence, and distribution of condoms in schools. Available at: www.ama-assn.org/apps/pf_new/pf_online?f_n=resultLink&doc=policyfiles/HnE/H-170.968.HTM&s_t=abstinence&catg=AMA/HnE&catg=AMA/BnGnC&catg=AMA/DIR&&nth=1&&st_p=0&nth=2&. Accessed April 26, 2007

55. Kittredge D. Abstinence and abstinence-only education. *J Adolesc Health*. 2006;39:150–151
56. Elster A, Fleming M. Abstinence and abstinence-only education. *J Adolesc Health*. 2006;39:150
57. Kirby D, Rolleri L, Wilson M. *Tool to Assess the Characteristics of Effective Sex and STD/HIV Education Programs*. Washington, DC: Healthy Teen Network; 2007
58. Solomon J, Card JJ. *Making the List: Understanding, Selecting, and Replicating Effective Teen Pregnancy Prevention Programs*. Washington, DC: National Campaign to Prevent Teen Pregnancy; 2004

Sexual and Reproductive Health Care for Adolescents: Legal Rights and Policy Challenges

Abigail English, JD

Center for Adolescent Health & the Law, 310 Kildaire Road, Suite 100, Chapel Hill, NC 27516 USA

Laws developed over the past half-century have helped to make it possible for adolescents to receive essential sexual and reproductive health care.[1] Those who wrote these laws recognized that many adolescents engage in some form of sexual activity before they reach the age of adulthood[2] and that access to appropriate health care is necessary to protect their health and further the public health. Responding to the reality that some adolescents will not seek sexual and reproductive health care unless they can do so on a confidential basis, the laws allow many adolescents of the age of minority to give their own consent, protect confidentiality, and provide financial support for the care.[3,4] A majority of adolescents do share information with their parents about health care concerns, even sensitive ones related to sexual activity,[5] and parents unquestionably have a significant role to play in protecting the sexual and reproductive health of adolescents. Nevertheless, the laws that allow minors to give their consent for and receive confidential care also play an important role in the effective delivery of sexual and reproductive health services to the adolescents who need them.[3,4]

The legal framework for consent and confidentiality in adolescent health care is embodied in federal and state constitutions, statutes enacted by legislatures, regulations promulgated by administrative agencies, and cases decided by courts.[6,7] The consent requirements for adolescents to receive health care are contained primarily in state court decisions and in statutes known as state minor consent laws.[8] Confidentiality protections for adolescents' health information are often contained in these minor consent laws, the federal medical privacy regulations known as the Health Insurance Portability and Accountability Act (HIPAA) Privacy Rule, and in state medical privacy laws.[8,9] Other significant laws include statutes that provide for the emancipation of minors, court decisions that delineate the mature-minor doctrine, regulations that protect adolescents'

---

*Corresponding author.
E-mail address: english@cahl.org (A. English).

access to confidential family planning services in publicly funded programs, and court decisions that interpret the constitutional right of privacy.[8]

SEXUAL AND REPRODUCTIVE HEALTH CARE NEEDS

Adolescents' needs for sexual and reproductive health care encompass a broad and diverse range of services. They include, among others, contraceptive counseling, services, and supplies; pregnancy testing, counseling, and referral; abortion services, including counseling, referral, and termination of pregnancy; prenatal, maternity, and postpartum care; sexually transmitted disease (STD) prevention, testing, diagnosis, and treatment; HIV prevention, testing, diagnosis, and treatment; counseling about sexual orientation; and care related to sexual assault and abuse.[6]

Often the terms "reproductive health care" or "family planning services" are used loosely and refer to 1 or more of the above-listed services without clearly indicating the scope of the term's intended meaning. In some contexts, a term such as "family planning services" will have a specific technical meaning or legal definition. In addition, although it is important to understand the full scope of sexual and reproductive health services that adolescents might need, many of the laws that affect the delivery of these services relate to 1 or more specific services rather than the entire scope of these services.

It is also important to understand that although some adolescents seek sexual and reproductive health care directly by going to a family planning clinic for contraceptives or to a health department for STD testing, it is often a visit for another purpose such as a sports physical or an acute care need that serves as a gateway to services to address sexual and reproductive health needs.[7,10] Therefore, adolescents' access to sexual and reproductive health care may depend significantly on their access to health care in general, and the relevant laws concerning consent, confidentiality, and the financing of care must be understood in this context.

ROLE OF CONFIDENTIALITY

Research has often shown that confidentiality protections can increase the likelihood that adolescents will receive needed health care and that privacy concerns can limit access to essential care.[5,11-19] Adolescents have reported specific concerns about whether their parents will be informed, and study findings have shown that these concerns can have an effect on their use of health care.[5,11-13] Concerns about privacy can lead adolescents to delay seeking health care or forgo it entirely[13] and can affect their choice of provider,[17,20] their candor in responding to questions about sensitive topics,[18] and their acceptance of certain interventions such as pelvic examinations and testing for STDs and HIV.[21-23]

The delays and foregone care associated with the loss of confidentiality may also result in increased adolescent pregnancies and STDs, along with the associated economic costs.[24,25]

Health care professional organizations have recognized the key role that confidentiality can play in ensuring that adolescents receive the care they need and have adopted ethical codes, policy statements, and practice guidelines that support the provision of confidential care to this age group.[26,27] These policies and ethical principles address both the general need for protecting confidentiality in heath care and the importance of addressing the particular needs for confidential services among adolescents who are sexually active.[26] Consistent with both the evidence gained from research and the guidance provided by health care professional organizations, laws and policies have been put in place over the past half-century that enable adolescents to receive confidential sexual and reproductive health services.[1,3,4]

CONSENT FOR CARE

Adolescents who are over the age of majority are considered to be adults and can give their own consent for health care.[28,29] For an adolescent who is under the age of 18, which is the age of majority, the consent of a parent or a legal guardian is generally required.[28,29] However, numerous exceptions to this basic rule allow care to be provided without the consent of a parent.[28,29]

Depending on the specific circumstances, consent for a minor's care may be provided by a legal guardian, a court, or even a foster parent or other adult caretaker.[28,29] Also, in emergencies, care may be provided without the previous consent of a parent, although the health care provider is usually required to inform the parent as soon as possible.[28,29]

The laws that authorize minors to give their own consent for health care are, for the most part, state laws.[8] States began to enact specific statutes to enable minors to obtain care without parental consent, beginning in the middle of the 20th century.[1] Over the next half-century, every state enacted some of these statutes, which are generally grouped into 2 broad categories: laws that are based on the status of the minor and those that are based on the type of care the minor is seeking.[8]

Within each of these broad categories, some of the laws contain additional variations. For example, a law may contain 1 or more of the following elements: an age limit, a limit on the range of specific services covered, or enumeration of the providers or sites that may deliver the care.[8] In addition, a law may contain a statement that a physician or other health care professional may, in good faith, rely on representations made by the minor that he or she is legally allowed to consent.[8] Also, a law may specify whether the parent or the minor is financially responsible for payment when the minor does give his or her consent. Finally, a law may include specific provisions regarding whether information about the care for which the minor gives his or her consent may be disclosed to parents or guardians.[8]

Every state has enacted 1 or more statutes that allow minors to consent for health care based on their status. The most common status categories in which states have laws that expressly allow minors to consent for health care include emancipated minors, minors who are living apart from their parents (including homeless and runaway youth), minors who are married, minors who are pregnant, and minors who are parents.[8] In addition, there are other categories in which a small number of states have laws that allow minors to consent for health care, such as those who are in the military or are incarcerated.[8] When minors are allowed to consent for health care on the basis of their status, they usually are able to consent to all types of care, including sexual and reproductive health care, unless there is a specific limitation in the law.[8] The most common exceptions are for abortion, which may require parental consent or notification or a court order, and for sterilization, which is generally precluded for minors without a court order.[8]

Every state has enacted 1 or more statutes that allow minors to consent for specific types of health care. The most common categories of care for which states have laws that expressly allow minors to consent are emergency care, general medical care, family planning services or contraceptive care, pregnancy-related care, STD/venereal disease care, reportable-disease care, HIV/AIDS care, drug or alcohol counseling or treatment, and outpatient mental health services.[8,30-32] A few states allow minors to consent for other services such as bone marrow transplantation or care related to sexual assault.[8]

The concept of the "mature minor" is familiar to many health care professionals who treat adolescents, but its origin and meaning are not always well understood. The mature-minor doctrine was developed as the result of court decisions. Generally, according to the mature-minor doctrine, a physician is not liable if he or she provides care without parental consent when the care is within the mainstream of medical opinion, is not of a high-risk variety, and is provided in a nonnegligent manner, as long as the minor is an older adolescent who is capable of giving informed consent to the care and does voluntarily consent.[28]

The doctrine has been expressly accepted or favorably discussed by courts in several states.[33,34] Many fewer states have expressly rejected the doctrine's validity. The doctrine is often relied on as a justification for accepting the informed consent of mature minors for health care, even in states in which courts have not expressly accepted the doctrine.[6-8,28]

The concept of the mature minor has also been acknowledged, although without specific definition, in US Supreme Court cases in which rulings on requirements for parental consent or notification for a minor to obtain an abortion have been made.[35] Also, it is often mentioned in court cases in which the right of a minor to obtain an abortion without parental consent or notification through a state's judicial bypass procedure has been addressed.[35]

Only a few states have incorporated the mature-minor doctrine into a statute. For example, a small number of states have enacted statutes that allow minors to give their own consent for care if they have "sufficient intelligence to understand and appreciate the consequences of the proposed surgical or medical treatment or procedures," and this type of legal language (or language similar to it) has been used.[8]

PROTECTION OF CONFIDENTIALITY

Numerous laws protect the confidentiality of health care information, and many of these laws apply to adolescents who are minors and to adults. These laws include the constitutional right of privacy, minor consent laws, medical records and health privacy laws, evidentiary privileges, and funding statutes, among others.[6–8]

In almost every state, the minor consent laws contain 1 or more provisions that address confidentiality or disclosure of information when a minor is allowed to give consent for care.[8] In a few states, either the minor consent laws or the medical privacy laws specify that when a minor has consented to care, information about the care may not be disclosed without the permission of the minor.[8] In some states, a general disclosure provision applies to all of the minor consent laws; in others, a specific disclosure provision is included within 1 or more, but not all, of the minor consent laws.[8] Thus, the disclosure provisions are not necessarily consistent among different services, even within the same state. Most of the disclosure provisions address the circumstances under which a health care provider may disclose information to a parent when a minor has consented to the care.[8] These disclosure provisions are of particular importance in light of the HIPAA Privacy Rule.

The most important development in recent years that affects the confidentiality of adolescents' health care information is embodied in the federal medical privacy regulations known as the HIPAA Privacy Rule, which was issued under the Health Insurance Portability and Accountability Act of 1996.[9] The rule created new rights for individuals to have access to their protected health information and to control the disclosure of that information in some circumstances. It contains specific requirements that affect medical charts and information pertaining to the care of minors.[9] The HIPAA Privacy Rule provides, in general, that when minors legally consent to health care or can receive it without parental consent, or when a parent has assented to an agreement of confidentiality between the minor and the health care provider, the parent does not necessarily have an automatic right to access the minor's health information. That right to access depends on state laws or other applicable laws.[9]

Thus, a health care provider must look to state laws or other laws to determine if they specifically address the confidentiality of a minor's health information.[9] State or other laws that explicitly require, permit, or prohibit disclosure of information to a parent are controlling.[9] If state or other laws are silent on the question of parents' access, a health care professional exercising professional judgment has discretion to determine whether to grant access.[9] The relevant sources of state or other laws that a health care provider must consider when deciding whether to disclose information about a minor's sexual and reproductive health care include state minor consent laws, state medical privacy laws, the federal confidentiality rules for the federal Title X Family Planning Program, and court cases that interpret both these laws and the constitutional right of privacy.[8,9,36]

SPECIAL CONSENT AND CONFIDENTIALITY CONSIDERATIONS FOR SEXUAL AND REPRODUCTIVE HEALTH CARE

Special considerations apply to consent and confidentiality questions that pertain to family planning, contraception, and pregnancy-related care for minors. In addition to the explicit provisions of state minor consent laws, many of the most important considerations are articulated in court decisions on the basis of the constitutional right of privacy and the confidentiality requirements that are part of the federal Title X Family Planning Program and Medicaid.

Of note is that every state allows minors to consent to diagnosis and treatment for STDs.[8,32] Moreover, in every state, it should be possible for minors to receive contraceptive services and other pregnancy-related care on the basis of their own consent.[37,38] The vast majority of states have an explicit statute that allows minors to consent for these services.[8,30] Even without an explicit statute, however, minors should be able to consent on the basis of the mature-minor rule or the constitutional right of privacy and can do so at sites that are funded by the federal Title X Family Planning Program.[37,38]

In contrast to the prevailing policies for contraception, prenatal care, and STD care, most states have statutes that require either parental consent or notification for minors to obtain an abortion unless they have obtained a court order through a legal proceeding generally known as a judicial bypass.[39,40] In a few states, courts have found parental consent or notification requirements for abortion unconstitutional on the basis of the right of privacy in the state constitution.[6,7] However, even in such states, continued attempts are made to override these court decisions and impose a requirement of parental involvement by altering the content of the statute or adopting the requirement via a ballot referendum.

The US Supreme Court has held that the constitutional right of privacy extends to minors and adults and that it encompasses minors' reproductive decisions.[35,41] The Supreme Court has also explicitly recognized that minors' access to contraceptives falls within the ambit of the constitutional right of privacy.[42] Moreover, courts have not found that parental consent for minors to obtain contraceptives is required and have struck down laws that attempted to require parental consent or notification for contraceptives in several cases.[43–47] Therefore, even in the absence of a statute that authorizes minors to consent for family planning services or contraceptive care, if there is no valid statute or case prohibiting them from doing so, it would be reasonable to conclude that minors may give their own consent for these services.[37] This conclusion would also be consistent with the mature-minor doctrine.[37]

In every state, at sites that receive funds under the federal Title X Family Planning Program, minors are legally able to obtain family planning services and contraceptive care without parental consent or notification.[1,7,37] Title X specifies that family planning services must be available without regard to age and includes detailed confidentiality rules.[7,8] Title X encourages, but does not require, family participation.[7,8] The Medicaid program also requires confidential family planning services to be available to adolescents and adults who are eligible for Medicaid.[8,48]

FINANCIAL ACCESS

A critical factor for whether adolescents receive the sexual and reproductive health services they need is the availability of a source of payment for the services. Although a significant majority of adolescents have private health insurance coverage, a growing number are publicly insured under Medicaid or the State Children's Health Insurance Program (SCHIP); however, millions remain uninsured.[49] Adolescents with private health insurance coverage usually cannot use it for sexual and reproductive health services that they need on a confidential basis, because documentation of services is almost always sent to the policyholder, who is either a parent or another adult family member.[50]

Thus, even some adolescents with private health insurance rely on public programs; particularly, the federal Title X Family Planning Program.[7] Not only does Title X require confidential family planning services to be available without regard to age, it also ensures that when minors apply for services, their financial eligibility should be determined by reference solely to their own financial circumstances and not that of their parents or other family members.[1,37] Thus, as a legal matter, minors do not encounter financial barriers when they seek confidential services from Title X–funded clinics.

For adolescents with public health insurance, Medicaid and SCHIP can provide coverage for a significant scope of sexual and reproductive health services.[10,51] Medicaid has long been a significant source of financing for reproductive health services for low-income women and children in the United States and continues to assume increasing importance. The Medicaid benefit package includes coverage for a broad range of reproductive health services, and other services that address sexual and reproductive health needs, and adolescent Medicaid beneficiaries are entitled to receive the full range of these covered services.[10] Many of the services that adolescents need to meet their reproductive needs are not explicitly designated as reproductive health services but, nonetheless, are covered by Medicaid.[10,51] They include physician, hospital, clinic, laboratory, and radiograph services.[10] Other covered services are more explicitly for reproductive needs. They include family planning services and supplies and abortions, when necessary, to save the life of the mother or to end a pregnancy caused by rape or incest.[10,51] Medicaid law contains provisions designed to make family planning services accessible. For example, the federal matching rate for family planning services is 90%. Cost sharing may not be applied to family planning services, and beneficiaries must be allowed a free choice of family planning provider, even when they are enrolled in managed care plans that otherwise restrict choice of provider.[10,51] Moreover, Medicaid family planning services must be available to eligible minors who can be considered to be sexually active.[10]

In addition to Title X, Medicaid, and SCHIP, other publicly funded programs that help support sexual and reproductive health services that are available to adolescents include the Maternal and Child Health Block Grant and the Title XX Social Services Program.[51] The combination of private and public health insurance and other publicly funded programs such as Title X family planning provide a patchwork of financial support for the sexual and reproductive health care that adolescents need, although many adolescents slip through the cracks and do not have access.

CONCLUSIONS

A significant legal framework has been put in place since the middle of the 20th century that includes laws related to consent, confidentiality, and financial access. This legal framework has significantly improved adolescents' access to essential sexual and reproductive health care. Nevertheless, these important laws are frequently placed at risk and are subjected to efforts, both direct and indirect, to undermine their effectiveness. The risks include attempts to limit minor consent laws and restrict confidentiality protection by requiring parental consent or notification not only for abortion but also for contraception and STD care.[24,25] They also include measures, such as requirements for the reporting of adolescents' consensual sexual activity, that would discourage adolescents from seeking care and jeopardize both their access to care and their health.[52,53] Substantial additional risks are posed by the pressure in the federal budget to limit funding increases, even in programs such as the Title X Family Planning Program, that have been funded at essentially the same level for many years, despite substantial increases in need. An important challenge for those who want to promote the sexual and reproductive health of adolescents will be to preserve the legal framework that has developed over the last half-century by exposing efforts to dismantle it and to promote adequate financial support for the essential sexual and reproductive health care that adolescents need.

REFERENCES

1. English A, Morreale M. A legal and policy framework for adolescent health care: past, present, and future. *Houst J Health Law Policy*. 2001;1:63–108
2. Auslander BA, Rosenthal SL, Blythe MJ. Understanding sexual behaviors of adolescents within a biopsychosocial framework. *Adolesc Med*. 2007;18:434–448
3. English A, Ford CA. More evidence supports the need to protect confidentiality in adolescent health care. *J Adolesc Health*. 2007;40:199–200
4. Ford CA, English A. Limiting confidentiality of adolescent health services: what are the risks? *JAMA*. 2002;288:752–753
5. Jones RK, Purcell A, Singh S, Finer LB. Adolescents' reports of parental knowledge of adolescents' use of sexual health services and their reactions to parental notification for prescription contraception. *JAMA*. 2005;293:340–348
6. English A, Simmons PS. Legal issues in reproductive health care for adolescents. *Adolesc Med*. 1999;10:181–194
7. English A. Reproductive health services for adolescents: critical legal issues. *Obstet Gynecol Clin North Am*. 2000;27:195–211
8. English A, Kenney, KE. *State Minor Consent Laws: A Summary*. 2nd ed. Chapel Hill, NC: Center for Adolescent Health and the Law; 2003
9. English A, Ford CA. The HIPAA privacy rule and adolescents: legal questions and clinical challenges. *Perspect Sex Reprod Health*. 2004;36:80–86
10. English A, Morreale M, Stinnett A. *Adolescents in Public Health Insurance Programs: Medicaid and CHIP*. Chapel Hill, NC: Center for Adolescent Health and the Law; 1999
11. Reddy DM, Fleming R, Swain C. Effect of mandatory parental notification on adolescent girls' use of sexual health care services. *JAMA*. 2002;288:710–714
12. Klein JD, Wilson KM, McNulty M, Kapphahn C, Collins KS. Access to medical care for adolescents: results from the 1997 Commonwealth Fund Survey of the Health of Adolescent Girls. *J Adolesc Health*. 1999;25:120–130
13. Ford C, Bearman P, Moody J. Foregone health care among adolescents. *JAMA*. 1999;82:2227–2234
14. Marks A, Malizio J, Hoch J, Brody R, Fisher M. Assessment of health needs and willingness to utilize health care resources of adolescents in a suburban population. *J Pediatr*. 1983;102:456–460
15. Zabin LS, Stark HA, Emerson MR. Reasons for delay in contraceptive clinic utilization: adolescent clinic and nonclinic populations compared. *J Adolesc Health*. 1991;12:225–232
16. Cheng TL, Savageau JA, Sattler AL, DeWitt TG. Confidentiality in health care: a survey of knowledge, perceptions, and attitudes among high school students. *JAMA*. 1993;269:1404–1407
17. Sugerman S, Halfon N, Fink A, Anerson M, Valle L, Brook RH. Family planning clinic clients: their usual health care providers, insurance status, and implications for managed care. *J Adolesc Health*. 2000;27:25–33
18. Ford CA, Millstein SG, Halpern-Felsher BL, Irwin CE Jr. Influence of physician confidentiality assurances on adolescents' willingness to disclose information and seek future health care a randomized controlled trial. *JAMA*. 1997;278:1029–1034
19. Lehrer JA, Pantell R, Tebb K, Shafer MA. Forgone health care among U.S. adolescents: associations between risk characteristics and confidentiality concern. *J Adolesc Health*. 2007; 40:218–226

20. Lane MA, McCright J, Garrett K, Millstein SG, Bolan G, Ellen JM. Features of sexually transmitted disease services important to African-American adolescents. *Arch Pediatr Adolesc Med.* 1999;153:829–833
21. Thrall JS, McCloskey L, Ettner SL, Rothman E, Tighe JE, Emans SJ. Confidentiality and adolescents' use of providers for health information and for pelvic exams. *Arch Pediatr Adolesc Med.* 2000;154:885–892
22. Ford CA, Best D, Miller WC. The pediatric forum: confidentiality and adolescents' willingness to consent to sexually transmitted disease testing. *Arch Pediatr Adolesc Med.* 2001;155:1072–1073
23. Meehan TM, Hansen H, Klein WC. The impact of parental consent on the HIV testing of minors. *Am J Public Health.* 1997;87:1338–1341
24. Franzini L, Marks E, Cromwell PF, et al. Economic cost due to health consequences of teen's loss of confidentiality in obtaining reproductive health care services in Texas. *Arch Pediatr Adolesc Med.* 2004;158:1182–1184
25. Zavodny M. Fertility and parental consent for minors to receive contraceptives. *Am J Public Health.* 2004;94:1347–1351
26. Morreale M, Stinnett AJ, Dowling EC, eds. *Policy Compendium on Confidential Health Services for Adolescents.* 2nd ed. Chapel Hill, NC: Center for Adolescent Health and the Law; 2005
27. Ford C, English A, Sigman G. Confidential health care for adolescents: a position paper of the Society for Adolescent Medicine. *J Adolesc Health.* 2004;35:160–167
28. Holder AR. *Legal Issues in Pediatric and Adolescent Medicine.* 2nd ed. New Haven, CT: Yale University Press; 1985
29. Rosovsky FA. *Consent to Treatment: A Practical Guide.* 3rd ed. Gaithersburg, MD: Aspen Publishers; 2001
30. Guttmacher Institute. State policies in brief: minors' access to contraceptive services as of October 1, 2007. Available at: http://guttmacher.org/statecenter/spibs/spib_MACS.pdf. Accessed October 7, 2007
31. Guttmacher Institute. State policies in brief: minors' access to prenatal care as of October 1, 2007. Available at: http://guttmacher.org/statecenter/spibs/spib_MAPC.pdf. Accessed October 7, 2007
32. Guttmacher Institute. State policies in brief: minors' access to STI services as of October 1, 2007. Available at: http://guttmacher.org/statecenter/spibs/spib_MASS.pdf. Accessed October 7, 2007
33. *Cardwell v Bechtol*, 724 SW 2d 739 (Tenn 1987)
34. *In the Interest of E.G.*, 515 NE 2d 287 (Ill App 1987)
35. *Bellotti v Baird*, 443 US 622 (1979)
36. Health Privacy Project. State health privacy laws (2nd edition, 2002). Available at: www.healthprivacy.org/info-url_nocat2304/info-url_nocat.htm. Accessed October 7, 2007
37. English A. *Contraceptive Services for Adolescents: What Health Care Providers Need to Know About the Law.* Chapel Hill, NC: Center for Adolescent Health and the Law and Washington, DC: Healthy Teen Network; 2006. Available at: www.cahl.org/PDFs/HelpingTeensStayHealthy&Save_Full%20Report.pdf. Accessed October 7, 2007
38. Paul EW, Klassel D. Minors' constitutional right to consent to contraceptive services: the limits of state power. *Women's Rights Law Reporter.* 1987;10:45–64
39. Guttmacher Institute. State policies in brief: parental involvement in minors' abortions as of October 1, 2007. Available at: http://guttmacher.org/statecenter/spibs/spib_PIMA.pdf. Accessed October 7, 2007
40. Crosby MC, English A. Mandatory parental involvement/judicial bypass laws: do they protect adolescents' health? *J Adolesc Health.* 1991;12:143–147
41. *Planned Parenthood of Central Missouri v Danforth*, 428 US 52 (1979)
42. *Carey v Population Services International*, 531 US 678 (1977)
43. *Doe v Irwin*, 615 F 2d 1162 (6th Cir 1980), *cert denied*, 449 US 829 (1980)
44. *New York v Heckler*, 719 F 2d 1191 (2d Cir 1983)
45. *Planned Parenthood Federation of America v Heckler*, 712 F 2d 650 (DC Cir 1983)
46. *Planned Parenthood Association of Utah v Matheson*, 582 F Supp 1001 (D Utah 1983)

47. *T.H. v Jones*, 425 F Supp 873 (D. Utah), *aff'd in part*, 425 US 986 (1976)
48. National Health Law Program. Medicaid coverage of reproductive health services. Available at: www.healthlaw.org/library.cfm?fa=download&resourceID=81369&print. Accessed October 7, 2007
49. Newacheck PW, Park MJ, Brindis CD, Biehl M, Irwin CE Jr. Trends in private and public health insurance for adolescents. *JAMA*. 2004;291:1231–1237
50. American Medical Association, Council on Scientific Affairs. Confidential health services for adolescents. *JAMA* 1993;269:1420–1424
51. National Conference of State Legislatures. Providing reproductive health services for adolescents: state options. Available at: www.ncsl.org/programs/health/forum/pub6768.htm. Accessed October 7, 2007
52. English A, Teare C. Statutory rape enforcement and child abuse reporting: effects on health care access for adolescents. *DePaul Law Rev*. 2001;50:827–864
53. Teare C, English A. Nursing practice and statutory rape: effects of reporting and enforcement on access to care for adolescents. *Nurs Clin North Am Adolesc Health*. 2002;37:393–404

A

Abstinence: definition of, 559
Abstinence-only education
  definition, 560
  ethical concerns, 565
  federal support for, 561, 564
  increase in, 562
  medical accuracy of, 564–565
  public support for, 561
Acanthuses Nigerians, 432
Acne, 431, 432
Adherence, to medical regimens, 550
Adolescent Sexual Orientation, **508–518**
Adrenal androgens, production of, 426
Adrenarche: definition, 426
Advertising
  of contraceptives, 497–498
  sexual content, 491–492
Anal intercourse, 439
Approaches to Adolescent Sexuality Education, **558–570**
Asexual orientation, 511
Asthma, 522, 523, 525

B

Biopsychosocial framework,
  understanding of sexual behaviors within, 434–448
Bisexual orientation, 449, 511, 512
Body-mass index (BMI), 430, 431
Bone age, 432
Breast development, stages of, 426–427, 429–430
Bullying, 531–532

C

Cervical cancer, 443, 552
CHCs. See *Chronic health conditions*.
Childhood cancer, 522

Chlamydia, 443, 524, 551
Chronic fatigue syndrome, 525
Chronic health conditions (CHCs), adolescents with
  cognitive functioning, 522–523
  guidance and counseling for sexual health, 524–525
  health risk behaviors, 519–520
  physical and psychosocial development, 520–521
  physical development and functioning, 521–522
  sexual health, 519–529
  social/development and emotional functioning, 523–524
Clinicians. See also *Pediatricians*.
  role of, in addressing adolescent sexuality, 548–549
Coercion, 533–534, 539–540
Cognitive functioning
  adolescents with CHCs, 522–523
"coming out," 515
Communication, parent-adolescent, 462–464
Comprehensive sexuality education
  definition, 560–561
  erosion of, 562
  federal support for, 561
  medical accuracy of, 564
  program effectiveness, 562–563
  public support for, 561
  selecting and adapting for a community, 566
Condom use
  in abstinence-only education, 560, 565
  in comprehensive sexuality education, 560
  in entertainment-education, 500
  parenting interventions, 465
  sexual behaviors and, 435, 437, 439, 440
Confidentiality
  of health care information, protection of, 575–576
  importance of, in evaluating sexual

orientation and behaviors, 513–514
role of, in health care, 574–575
special considerations for sexual and reproductive health care, 576–577
state laws, 545–546, 575–576

Congenital adrenal hyperplasia, 432

Consent for care, 573–577

Constitutional delay, 432

Contraception
in abstinence-only education, 560, 565
addressing in office setting, 553–554
advertising of contraceptives, 497–498
in comprehensive sexuality education, 560
emergency contraception, 500, 545, 554, 555
religiosity/spirituality and, 475–476

Counseling, for sexual health, adolescents with CHCs, 524–525

Cross-gender behavior, 512–513

Cystic fibrosis (CF), 520, 521, 525

D

Dating, 454, 455, 465, 534

Depression, 442, 443, 523, 541

Development of Intimate Relationships in Adolescence, **449–459**

Diabetes, 432, 520, 522, 523, 525

E

Early adolescence
counseling regarding sexuality, 547
development of intimate relationships, 450–452

Education, sexuality
approaches to, 558–570
definitions, 559–561
entertainment-education, 499–500
important issues in, 562–565
media-literacy education, 500–502
professional consensus statements and position papers, 565–566
sex-education landscape, 559–562

Emergency contraception, 500, 545, 554, 555

Emotional functioning, of adolescents with CHCs, 523–524

Entertainment-education, 499–500

Epilepsy, 521, 522

Ethical standards, in sexuality education, 565

F

Families
HPV vaccine and, 466
modeled behaviors, 464–465
role of, in addressing adolescent sexuality, 549

Federal support, for sexuality education, 561

Financial access, 577–578

From Calvin Klein to Paris Hilton and MySpace: Adolescents, Sex, and the Media, **484–507**

G

Gay youth. See also *Homosexual orientation*
intimacy development, 449

Gender identity, 511, 512–513

Gender-identity disorder, prevalence of, 513

Gender-identity dysphoria, criteria for, 512

Genital herpes, 438, 443

Gonadarche: definition, 426

Gonorrhea, 438, 443, 524

Growth velocity, 428, 430, 431

Guidance, for sexual health, adolescents with CHCs, 524–525

Gynecomastia, 431, 432

H

Harassment, sexual, 532–533

Health risk behaviors, in adolescents with CHCs, 519–529

Healthy sexual behavior, office-based interventions to promote, 544

Help-seeking behaviors, 538

Hemophilia, 523

Hepatitis B and C, 523, 552

Herpes simplex virus, 438, 443

Heterosexual orientation, 508–511

Homosexual orientation, 508–512

Hormonal contraceptive methods, 440, 553–555

Human immunodeficiency virus (HIV)
adolescents with CHCs, 523
anal intercourse and, 439
HIV/AIDS, 443, 488, 500
information access, 565
media content, 488–489, 500
prevention programs, 437, 562
risk-reduction intervention, 465
testing for, 572

Human papillomavirus (HPV)
infections, 443
vaccine, 466, 552

I

Immunizations, 466, 552

Infertility, 443, 525

Internet
impact on adolescents with CHCs, 523–524
pornography/sexually explicit media, 490–491

Interventions
media, for sexual health, potential of, 497–502
parenting interventions, 465

Intimate relationships, development of, 449–459
clinical implications, 456–457
in early adolescence, 450–452
influences on romantic relationships, 456
in late adolescence, 452–456

J

Juvenile idiopathic arthritis, 523–524, 525

K

Kissing, 435, 450, 551, 559

Knee injuries, 432

L

Late adolescence
counseling regarding sexuality, 548
development of intimate relationships, 452–456

Legal issues. See *Confidentiality; Consent for care*

Legal rights, in sexual and reproductive health care for adolescents, 571–581

Lesbian youth. See also *Homosexual orientation*
intimacy development, 449

M

Magazines, sexual content, 489

Masturbation, 435–437

Mature-minor doctrine, 574–575, 577

Media
adolescents' use of, 484–485
effects on teens' sexual behavior, 494
influence on sexual norms and scripts, 493–494
interventions, potential for sexual health, 497–502
learning about sex from, 492–497
media-literacy education, 500–502
pornography/sexually explicit media, 490–491
sexual content, 485–492
use and interpretation, differences in, 494–497

Medical accuracy, of sexuality education, 563–565

Medical needs, of sexually active patients, 550–555
contraception, 553–555
immunizations, 552
pelvic examinations, 524, 544, 550–551, 572
testing for and treating STIs, 551–552

Medroxyprogesterone (Depo Provera), 553, 554

Menarche: definition of, 426

Menstrual period, first, age of onset of, 426

Middle adolescence, counseling regarding sexuality, 547–548

Modeled behaviors in the family, 464–465

Monitoring, parental, 461–462

Mood swings, 523

Musculoskeletal problems, 431, 432

Music, sexual content, 489–490

Myopia, 431, 432

MySpace, 484

N

Neisseria gonorrhea, 551

Nocturnal emissions, 431

Non-gender-conforming youth. See also *Gender identity.*
intimacy development, 449

O

Office-Based Interventions to Promote Healthy Sexual Behavior, **544–557**

Opposite-gender friendships, 451–453

Oral contraceptive pills, 475, 476, 553

Oral sex, 437–439, 454, 551, 559

Outcomes, sexual health, religiosity/spirituality and, 476–478

"outercourse," 436–437

P

Parental Influences on Adolescent Sexual Behaviors, **460–470**
families and the HPV vaccine, 466
modeled behaviors in the family, 464–465
parent-adolescent communication, 462–464
parental monitoring, 461–462
parenting interventions, 465

Pediatricians, role of, in sexuality education programs, 567

Peers, role of, in addressing adolescent sexuality, 549

Pelvic examinations, 524, 544, 550–551, 572

Pelvic inflammatory disease, 443

Physical development and functioning, of adolescents with CHCs, 520–522

Physical health risks, sexual orientation and, 510–511

Policy challenges, sexual and reproductive health care for adolescents, 571–581

Polycystic ovary syndrome, 432, 521

Pornography, 490–491

Posttraumatic stress disorder, 539

Preadolescents, counseling regarding sexuality, 547

Pregnancy/birth rates and trends, 442–443, 559

Professional consensus statements and position papers, 565–566

Program effectiveness
abstinence-only programs, 563
comprehensive sexuality programs, 562–563

Psychological health risks, sexual orientation and, 510–511

Psychosocial development, influences of CHCs on, 520–521

Pubarche: definition, 426

Puberty, **425–433**
adolescents with CHCs, 521–522
common medical issues associated with, 431–432
early or late, 431–432, 434, 521
sequence and timing of, 426–431

Pubic hair, stages, 426, 428–431

Public support, for sexuality education, 561

R

Reality TV, sexual content, 488

Relationship Violence in Adolescence, **530–543**

Religiosity, Spirituality, and Adolescent Sexuality, **471–483**

Religious/spiritual factors
contraception and, 475–476
definitions and measurement of, 472–473
programs/clinical implications, 478–480
relation to sexual health outcomes, 476–478
sexual behaviors/attitudes and, 473–475

Reproductive behavior, 558–570

Reproductive health care. See *Sexual and reproductive health care.*

Romantic relationships, influences on, 456

S

Safe-sex behaviors, 437, 488

Scientific accuracy, of sexuality education, 563–565

Screening and counseling
  adolescent sexuality, 547–548
  sexual health, adolescents with CHCs, 524–525
  sexual orientation, 513–516

Sex education. see *Education, sexuality.*

Sex-reassignment surgery, 513

Sexual and reproductive health care
  consent for care, 573–577
  financial access, 577–578
  legal rights and policy challenges, 571–581
  needs, 572
  protection of confidentiality, 575–576
  role of confidentiality, 572–573
  special consent and confidentiality considerations, 576–577

Sexual and Reproductive Health Care for Adolescents: Legal Rights and Policy Challenges, **571–581**

Sexual attitudes, religiosity/spirituality and, 473–475

Sexual attraction, 484, 511–513

Sexual behavior(s)
  anal intercourse, 439
  approaches to adolescent sexuality education, 558–570
  gender identity and, 511–513
  masturbation, 435–437
  media's effects on, 494
  negative consequences of, 442–443
  oral sex, 437–439, 454
  parental influences on, 460–470
  religiosity/spirituality and, 473–475
  understanding of, within biopsychosocial framework, 434–448
  vaginal sexual intercourse, 440–441

Sexual health. See also *Sexual and reproductive health care.*
  adolescents with CHCs, 519–529
  media campaigns, 498–409
  religiosity/spirituality and, 476–478

Sexual Health of Adolescents With Chronic Health Conditions, **519–529**

Sexual identity
  attraction and behavior, 511–512
  development of, 509–510
  screening and counseling, 513–516

Sexually explicit media, 490–491

Sexually transmitted infections (STIs)
  adolescents with CHCs, 520, 522–525
  behaviors associated with spread of, 438–439
  prevention, 437, 444, 525, 547
  rates and trends, 443
  screening, 524, 547
  sexuality education programs, 558, 565
  testing for and treating, 550–552, 572, 576

Sexual orientation, 508–518
  development of sexual identity, 509–510
  gender identity, 511–513
  office-based interventions, 549–550
  psychological and physical health risks, 510–511
  screening and counseling, 513–516

Sexual violence, 535–538

Short stature, 431, 432

Soap operas, sexual content, 488–489

Social development
  adolescents with CHCs, 523–524

STIs. See *Sexually transmitted infections.*

Suicidal ideation and behavior, sexual orientation and, 510–511

Syphilis, 438

T

Tanner stages, 426

Television, sexual content, 485–488

Testicular volume, 428, 430, 521

Thelarche: definition, 426

Transgender youth
  gender identity, 512
  intimacy development, 449
  screening and counseling, 513–516

Transsexual individuals, 512, 513

U

Understanding Sexual Behaviors of Adolescents Within a Biopsychosocial Framework, **434–448**

V

Vaginal sexual intercourse, 440–441

Verbal and physical violence, 534–535

Violence, interpersonal, times of risk for, 450–452

Violence, relationship, 530–543
  bullying, 531–532
  clinical implications, 540–542
  coercion, 533–534, 539–540
  help-seeking behaviors, 538
  risk factors, 538
  sequelae, 538–540
  sexual harassment, 532–533
  sexual violence, 535–538
  verbal and physical violence, 534–535

Virginity status, 437